Ulnar-sided Wrist Pain

Editor

DAWN LAPORTE

HAND CLINICS

www.hand.theclinics.com

Consulting Editor
KEVIN C. CHUNG

November 2021 • Volume 37 • Number 4

ELSEVIER

1600 John F. Kennedy Boulevard • Suite 1800 • Philadelphia, Pennsylvania, 19103-2899

http://www.theclinics.com

HAND CLINICS Volume 37, Number 4
November 2021 ISSN 0749-0712, ISBN-13: 978-0-323-81327-3

Editor: Lauren Boyle
Developmental Editor: Hannah Almira Lopez

Hand Clinics (ISSN 0749-0712) is published quarterly by Elsevier Inc., 360 Park Avenue South, New York, NY 10010-1710. Months of publication are February, May, August, and November. Business and Editorial Offices: 1600 John F. Kennedy Blvd., Ste. 1800, Philadelphia, PA 19103-2899. Customer Service Office: 3251 Riverport Lane, Maryland Heights, MO 63043. Periodicals postage paid at New York, NY and at additional mailing offices. Subscription price is $439.00 per year (domestic individuals), $1039.00 per year (domestic institutions), $100.00 per year (domestic students/residents), $501.00 per year (Canadian individuals), $1086.00 per year (Canadian institutions), $562.00 per year (international individuals), $1086.00 per year (international institutions), $256.00 (international students/residents), and $100.00 (Canadian students/residents). Foreign air speed delivery is included in all *Clinics* subscription prices. All prices are subject to change without notice. **POSTMASTER:** Send address changes to *Hand Clinics*, Elsevier Health Sciences Division, Subscription Customer Service, 3251 Riverport Lane, Maryland Heights, MO 63043. Customer Service (orders, claims, online, change of address): Elsevier Health Sciences Division, Subscription **Customer Service, 3251 Riverport Lane, Maryland Heights, MO 63043. Tel: 1-800-654-2452 (U.S. and Canada); 314-447-8871 (outside U.S. and Canada). Fax: 314-447-8029. E-mail: journalscustomerservice-usa@elsevier.com (for print support); journalsonlinesupport-usa@elsevier.com (for online support).**

Reprints. For copies of 100 or more of articles in this publication, please contact the Commercial Reprints Department, Elsevier Inc., 360 Park Avenue South, New York, New York 10010-1710. Tel.: 212-633-3874; Fax: 212-633-3820; E-mail: reprints@elsevier.com.

Hand Clinics is covered in *MEDLINE/PubMed (Index Medicus), Current Contents/Clinical Medicine, EMBASE/Excerpta Medica,* and *ISI/BIOMED.*

Contributors

CONSULTING EDITOR

KEVIN C. CHUNG, MD, MS
Charles B. G. de Nancrede Professor of
Surgery, Professor of Plastic Surgery and
Orthopaedic Surgery, Chief of Hand Surgery,
Michigan Medicine, Assistant Dean for Faculty
Affairs, Associate Director of Global REACH,
University of Michigan Medical School, Ann
Arbor, Michigan, USA

EDITOR

DAWN LAPORTE, MD
Professor, Vice Chairman Education,
Department of Orthopaedic Surgery, Johns
Hopkins School of Medicine, Baltimore,
Maryland, USA

AUTHORS

JULIE ADAMS, MD
Professor, Department of Orthopaedic
Surgery, University of Tennessee College of
Medicine, Chattanooga, Tennessee, USA

YASMIN ALFAKI
Johns Hopkins University, Baltimore,
Maryland, USA

DONALD S. BAE, MD
Clinical Chief of Orthopedic Surgery, Boston
Children's Hospital, Professor of Orthopedic
Surgery, Harvard Medical School, Boston,
Massachusetts, USA

BRANDON BOYD, MD
Hand and Upper Extremity Fellow, Philadelphia
Hand to Shoulder Center, Philadelphia,
Pennsylvania, USA

MARION BURNIER, MD
Hand and Upper Extremity Surgical Institute,
Clinique du Medipole-Lyon, Villeurbanne,
France

JACQUELINE N. BYRD, MD, MPH
Research Fellow, Section of Plastic Surgery,
Department of Surgery, University of Michigan
Medical School, Ann Arbor, Michigan, USA;
Resident, Department of Surgery, The
University of Texas Southwestern Medical
School, Dallas, Texas, USA

KEVIN C. CHUNG, MD, MS
Charles B. G. de Nancrede Professor of
Surgery, Professor of Plastic Surgery and
Orthopaedic Surgery, Chief of Hand Surgery,
Michigan Medicine, Assistant Dean for Faculty
Affairs, Associate Director of Global REACH,
University of Michigan Medical School, Ann
Arbor, Michigan, USA

SAMUEL COHEN-TANUGI, MD
Atrium Health Department of Orthopedic
Surgery, Charlotte, North Carolina, USA

SHADPOUR DEMEHRI, MD
Johns Hopkins Department of Musculoskeletal
Radiology, Baltimore, Maryland, USA

GINA FARIAS-EISNER, MD
Hand and Microvascular Surgery Fellow, Hand, Elbow and Shoulder Center at University of Washington Medical Center - Roosevelt, Seattle, Washington, USA

GREGORY K. FAUCHER, MD
Division of Hand Surgery, Assistant Professor, University of South Carolina School of Medicine Greenville, Prisma Health-Upstate, The Hand Center, Greenville, South Carolina, USA

RAYMOND GLENN GASTON, MD
Fellowship Director, OrthoCarolina Hand and Upper Extremity Fellowship, Professor and Chief of Hand Surgery, Department of Orthopedic Surgery, Atrium Health/Atrium Musculoskeletal Institute, Charlotte, North Carolina

CHARLES A. GOLDFARB, MD
Professor and Executive Vice Chair, Department of Orthopaedic Surgery, Washington University, St Louis, Missouri, USA

MAX HAERLE, MD
Professor, Centre for Hand and Plastic Surgery, Orthopedic Clinic Markgröningen, Markgröningen, Germany

NICHOLAS IANNUZZI, MD
Assistant Professor, Chief, Orthopaedic Surgery, Puget Sound VA, Department of Orthopaedics and Sports Medicine, Hand, Elbow and Shoulder Center at University of Washington Medical Center - Roosevelt, Seattle, Washington, USA

SANJEEV KAKAR, MD, FAOA
Professor of Orthopaedic Surgery, Departments of Orthopaedic Surgery and Clinical Anatomy, Mayo Clinic, Rochester, Minnesota, USA

R. TIMOTHY KREULEN, MD
Johns Hopkins Department of Orthopaedic Surgery, Baltimore, Maryland, USA

FLORIAN M. LAMPERT, MD
Centre for Hand and Plastic Surgery, Orthopedic Clinic Markgröningen, Markgröningen, Germany

DAWN LAPORTE, MD
Professor, Vice Chairman Education, Department of Orthopaedic Surgery, Johns Hopkins School of Medicine, Baltimore, Maryland, USA

STELLA J. LEE, MD
Orthopedic Surgeon, Department of Surgery, Anna Jaques Hospital, Newburyport, Massachusetts, USA

NICO LEIBIG, MD
Centre for Hand and Plastic Surgery, Orthopedic Clinic Markgröningen, Markgröningen, Germany

MARK CHRISTIAN MOODY, MD
Division of Hand Surgery, Clinical Instructor, University of South Carolina School of Medicine Greenville, Prisma Health-Upstate, The Hand Center, Greenville, South Carolina, USA

SURESH K. NAYAR, MD
Johns Hopkins Department of Orthopaedic Surgery, Baltimore, Maryland, USA

REMY V. RABINOVICH, MD
Hand/Upper Extremity Surgeon, New York Hand and Wrist Center – Northwell Health, New York, New York, USA

SARAH E. SASOR, MD
Assistant Professor, Department of Plastic Surgery, Medical College of Wisconsin, Wauwatosa, Wisconsin, USA

LAUREN M. SHAPIRO, MD, MS
Fellow, Department of Orthopaedic Surgery, Duke University, Durham, North Carolina, USA

ANDREA TIAN, MD
Resident, Department of Orthopaedic Surgery, Washington University, St Louis, Missouri, USA

JEFFREY YAO, MD
Professor, Department of Orthopaedic Surgery, Stanford University, Redwood City, North Carolina, USA

DAVID S. ZELOUF, MD
Hand/Upper Extremity Surgeon, Philadelphia
Hand to Shoulder Center and Thomas
Jefferson University Hospitals, Philadelphia,
Pennsylvania, USA

STEPHEN D. ZOLLER, MD
Hand and Microvascular Surgery Fellow, Hand,
Elbow and Shoulder Center at University of
Washington Medical Center - Roosevelt,
Seattle, Washington, USA

Contents

 Video content accompanies this article at http://www.hand.theclinics.com.

comparative outcomes studies are limited, long-term retrospective outcome studies of TFCC repair and reconstructive techniques demonstrate improvement in pain, stability, range of motion, and disability.

Unsuccessful triangular fibrocartilage complex (TFCC) repair or reconstruction is poorly defined, often stemming from multiple causes, both patient and surgeon-related. Complete evaluation of the patient's psychosocial status and involvement in any litigation claims is essential, as is a thorough history, physical examination, and imaging workup to accurately diagnose TFCC injury, along with any concomitant wrist pathology. Awareness of common complications and technical errors is critical, and preventive treatment strategies should be implemented to minimize these events.

Triangular fibrocartilage complex (TFCC) tears can cause ulnar-sided wrist pain in children and adolescents following acute rotational injury or prior distal radius fracture. Surgical treatment, guided by the Palmer classification, is considered after activity modification and occupational therapy. All concomitant wrist pathologies, such as distal radioulnar joint instability, ulnocarpal impaction, and distal radius malunion, must be recognized and addressed at the time of TFCC debridement or repair. This article reviews recent literature guiding clinical evaluation and surgical treatment of children and adolescents with TFCC injuries. The authors' techniques for arthroscopic-assisted outside-in repair of Palmer 1B and 1D tears are described.

The use of wrist arthroscopy has evolved to being a powerful tool to not only diagnose but also treat wrist disorders. With the improvement in technology and surgical technique, many of the procedures can be done using dry wrist arthroscopy (DWA). DWA can be used to treat a wide spectrum of ulnar wrist disorders. In this article, we aim to highlight some technical pearls as well as show its use to treat common ulnar wrist pain disorders.

Lunotriquetral (LT) ligament injuries are uncommon, however, should be considered in patients with ulnar-sided wrist pain. LT injuries are often associated with other injuries but can occur in isolation. Understanding the anatomy and pathomechanics will aid in making the diagnosis. Similar to other injuries, a thorough history and focused physical examination is critical. Radiographs may show normal findings; however, advanced imaging can support the diagnosis. Arthroscopy remains the gold standard for diagnosis. Most patients do well with conservative management; however, injury acuity and severity will direct surgical management. Anatomy, pathophysiology, and treatment options are discussed.

HAND CLINICS

SERIES OF RELATED INTEREST:

Clinics in Plastic Surgery
https://www.plasticsurgery.theclinics.com/

Orthopedic Clinics of North America
https://www.orthopedic.theclinics.com/

Physical Medicine and Rehabilitation Clinics of North America
https://www.pmr.theclinics.com/

THE CLINICS ARE AVAILABLE ONLINE!
Access your subscription at:
www.theclinics.com

Preface

Current Innovations and Challenges in Ulnar-sided Wrist Pain

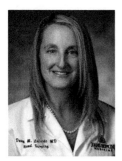

Dawn LaPorte, MD
Editor

Ulnar-sided wrist pain is one of the most vexing diagnostic and treatment challenges in hand surgery, due in part to the complexity of the associated anatomy and the multitude of different treatment options. There are many potential causes for ulnar-sided wrist pain, including trauma, sports, occupational injury, and overuse, and ulnar wrist pain can affect all age groups.

This issue of *Hand Clinics* shares expert perspectives on addressing challenges related to ulnar wrist pain, including nuances in diagnosis and imaging and controversies surrounding treatment: repair, reconstruction, and management of complications. Less-invasive treatment and earlier recovery may now be an option due to innovations in wrist arthroscopy. Discussion also includes differences in management of TFCC pathologic condition in adults compared with adolescents.

I am sincerely grateful to the authors of this issue, who are thought leaders in managing ulnar wrist pain, for sharing their wisdom and experience and advancing our understanding of this complex condition.

Dawn LaPorte, MD
Department of Orthopaedic Surgery
Johns Hopkins University School of Medicine
601 North Caroline Street
Baltimore, MD, 21287, USA

E-mail address:
dlaport1@jhmi.edu

https://doi.org/10.1016/j.hcl.2021.06.001
0749-0712/21/© 2021 Published by Elsevier Inc.

Examination of Ulnar-sided Wrist Pain

Samuel Cohen-Tanugi, MD[a], Raymond Glenn Gaston, MD[b,c],*

KEYWORDS

- Ulnar wrist pain • TFCC • ECU • Physical examination

KEY POINTS

- A broad differential diagnosis including traumatic and atraumatic causes of acute and chronic conditions is paramount to approaching ulnar wrist disorder.
- Understanding surface anatomy is critical for proper diagnosis of ulnar wrist pain.
- Specific provocative maneuvers can help differentiate between competing diagnoses of ulnar wrist pain.

 Video content accompanies this article at http://www.hand.theclinics.com.

The ulnar side of the wrist has historically been described as a black box to highlight the diagnostic challenge this anatomic region poses to many clinicians.[1–3] Ulnar-sided wrist pain is also commonly referred to as the back pain of hand surgery: a complaint that is ubiquitous, vague, and frustrating. When approaching this black box, it is best to first order a solid history and physical examination. An astute physical examination based on a thorough appreciation of the surface anatomy of the ulnar side of the wrist, coupled with a pointed history, can narrow the differential diagnosis, even before advanced imaging is obtained. Ulnar-sided wrist pain should resemble a puzzle in which a systematic approach will yield a definitive solution, rather than an impenetrable black box. To enable an accurate diagnosis, the clinician must first have a complete differential diagnosis: an exhaustive list of all of the structures present on the ulnar side of the wrist, including the osseous anatomy, ligaments, tendons, and neurovascular structures, with an understanding of the types of disorders that can affect each tissue type (**Box 1**). The next step is to gather relevant information from the patient's history to vastly narrow the differential diagnosis. Third, a thorough physical examination is performed. Observation, active and passive range of motion, and grip strength offer preliminary information, but the highest-yield diagnostic tool is the systematic palpation of all structures of the ulnar side of the wrist according to a confident understanding of the surface anatomy and comparison with the contralateral side. Once a particular diagnosis is suspected, specific provocative maneuvers can help differentiate similar complaints. If there is still uncertainty between disorders, differential injections into targeted structures in the office setting can be diagnostic and at times therapeutic.

CLINICAL HISTORY

Although this article concerns itself primarily with the physical examination of the ulnar side of the wrist, it is worth providing a brief overview of the most relevant aspects of a clinical history because it is critical in initially narrowing the differential diagnosis and provides crucial context to the examination. The history should focus on a few key questions.[4] Are the symptoms acute or chronic?

[a] Atrium Health Department Orthopedic Surgery, 1000 Blythe Boulevard, Charlotte, NC 28203, USA; [b] OrthoCarolina Hand and Upper Extremity Fellowship; [c] Department of Orthopedic Surgery, Atrium Health/Atrium Musculoskeletal Institute
* Corresponding author. OrthoCarolina Hand Center, 1915 Randolph Road, Charlotte, NC 28207.
E-mail address: Glenn.gaston@orthocarolina.com

Hand Clin 37 (2021) 467–475
https://doi.org/10.1016/j.hcl.2021.06.002

hand.theclinics.com

Box 1
Differential diagnosis of ulnar wrist pain by location

Fourth to fifth carpometacarpal joints

  Fracture

Base of fourth or fifth metacarpal

Dorsal shear fractures of hamate)

  Dislocation

  Arthritis (typically posttraumatic)

  Extensor carpi ulnaris insertional tendonitis

Lunotriquetral (LT) joint/ulnocarpal joint

  LT ligament tear

  Fracture

    Triquetrum (dorsal avulsion or body fracture)

    Lunate (body fracture or ligament avulsion)

  Proximal hamate arthrosis and LT tear

  Kienbock (avascular necrosis lunate)

  Incomplete coalition LT joint

  Ulnar impaction

  Triangular fibrocartilage complex (TFCC) tear

  Triquetrohamate impingement

Distal radioulnar joint

  Fracture

    Distal ulna

    Sigmoid notch radius

  Arthritis

  Instability

TFCC deep fiber tears

Ulnar styloid fracture

  ECU tendinosis/instability

Pisiform-triquetrum joint

  Fracture

  Arthritis

  Instability

  Insertional or calcific flexor carpi ulnaris tendonitis

Vascular causes

  Hypothenar hammer syndrome (ulnar artery pseudoaneurysm)

  Cardiac emboli

  Raynaud phenomenon or syndrome

  Peripheral vascular disease

  Thoracic outlet syndrome

Neurogenic causes

  Guyon canal (ganglion, hamate hook fracture, cycling, other mass effect)

  Cubital tunnel

  Neuroma

  C8 to T1 cervical radiculopathy

  Neurogenic thoracic outlet

  Lower brachial plexopathy

  Pancoast tumor

Was there antecedent trauma recently or in the past? For acute traumatic pain, clinicians should recognize classic injury patterns associated with specific activities. For instance, sports that involve gripping a bat or a club place the athletes at risk for a fracture of the hook of the hamate, which receives a direct blow such as during a so-called fat shot in golf, or a check swing in baseball.[5] Pain with a 2-handed backhand tennis swing often represents extensor carpi ulnaris (ECU) subsheath disorder.[6] Punching a wall raises concern for injury to the fourth and fifth metacarpals or carpometacarpal (CMC) joints. Ulnar-sided wrist pain after a car accident in which the steering wheel was being gripped at the time of impact, placing the wrists in extension and radial deviation, may lead to a lunotriquetral (LT) ligament tear.[7] For acute atraumatic pain, circumstances such as hours of gardening or chronic use of work tools point toward tendinous disorder. Acute symptoms associated with warmth and redness suggest inflammatory processes such as gout, infection, or calcific tendonitis. The language used to describe the nature of the pain can point toward a particular cause as well. For instance, inflammatory pain is more often described as hot and burning, compared with osteoarthritic pain which is described as persistent aches with episodes of sharp stabbing pain and stiffness in the morning.[8] Does the patient have other relevant medical conditions? It is important to keep systemic conditions in mind that can affect the distal extremities. A patient with an autoimmune condition (CREST [calcinosis, Raynaud phenomenon, esophageal dysmotility, sclerodactyly, and telangiectasia], Sjögren, and so forth) may also have Raynaud phenomenon. Rheumatoid arthritis can often present as tendonitis or tenosynovitis. Neurofibromatosis and peripheral nerve sheath tumors may affect the ulnar nerve anywhere along its course. Gout is the great mimicker and can affect the joints of the ulnar side of the wrist. A patient with endocarditis can send emboli into the small vessels of the hand.

In addition, it is critical to take note of any previous surgeries to the hand and wrist.

PHYSICAL EXAMINATION

The physical examination of the hand and wrist is conducted in a systematic fashion every time. It is worth remembering that, in addition to its diagnostic value, the physical examination constitutes an important ritual of care that is critical to the therapeutic relationship with the patient. The hand is a particularly intimate part of the body that is central to a person's identity. It is not by coincidence that, in his Ted Talk "A Doctor's Touch," physician-author Abraham Verghese describes starting his physical examination with a patient's hands.

For the entire examination, the examiner sits across from the patient, elbow resting on a surface and flexed at 90°, as if in preparation for an arm-wrestling match (**Fig. 1**). The examiner uses both hands to simultaneously stabilize the patient's forearm, wrist, and hand and perform the examination maneuvers. The first step should always be to ask the patient to point to the area of maximal pain and examine that location last. The examination then follows a stepwise sequence, starting with observation.

The appearance of the symptomatic hand and wrist should be compared with the unaffected side. Looking at the skin can indicate whether the patient has had previous surgery as shown by healed incisions, skin or nail conditions (ecchymosis, gouty tophi, onycholysis), or differential perfusion of the digits (eg, Raynaud). Comparing the shape of the hand and wrist with the contralateral side can reveal subtle deformities, such as a palmar sag of the carpus (seen in chronic and complete LT ligament tear), a prominent ulnar head (seen in chronic triangular fibrocartilage complex [TFCC] disruption, or caput ulnae), or swelling along the ulnar border of the distal forearm and wrist (tendinopathy/tenosynovitis). Altered position of the fingers and intrinsic muscle wasting may be signs of ulnar nerve disorder or other neurologic impairments (**Fig. 2**).

Range of motion of the wrist is performed first actively and then passively, measured with a goniometer, and compared with the contralateral side. Range of motion may be restricted, painful, or cause mechanical symptoms such as clicking, popping, or locking. Motor function of the ulnar nerve is easy to test alongside active range of motion. A thorough examination of ulnar nerve motor function includes testing key pinch to assess for Froment sign and Jeanne sign, as well as evaluating small finger adduction or Wartenberg sign. To test key pinch, the patient is asked to resist pulling a sheet of paper. Weakness of key pinch coupled with recruitment of the median nerve innervated flexor pollicis longus for thumb interphalangeal (IP) flexion to pinch is a positive Froment sign and indicates weakness of the adductor pollicis and first dorsal interosseus (**Fig. 3**). Jeanne sign, concomitant metacarpophalangeal (MP) hyperextension with key pinch, may also be noted in patients with ulnar nerve disorder. Wartenberg sign is the inability to maintain small finger adduction against the other fingers with

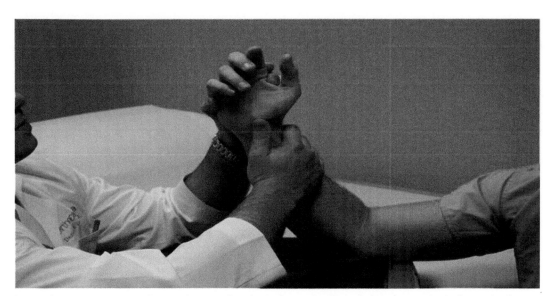

Fig. 1. The proper position for conducting the physical examination of the ulnar wrist is shown in the arm-wrestling position.

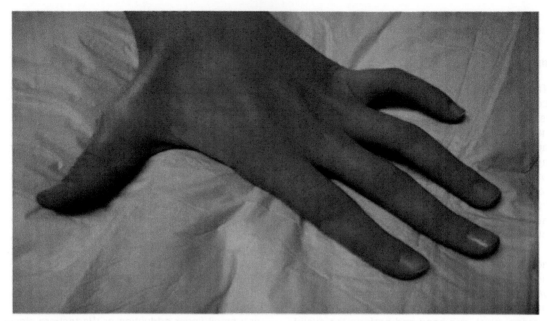

Fig. 2. A classic ulnar nerve palsy hand with intrinsic atrophy and clawing of the ulnar digits.

the hand placed flat on the table and indicates weakness of the third palmar interosseus with the extensor digiti minimi serving as the unopposed deformity force in the coronal plane. If ulnar nerve symptoms are present, whether sensory, motor, or both, the examination must include a full neurologic examination with particular attention paid to the Guyon canal as well as the cubital tunnel at the elbow. Disorder at Guyon canal and the cubital tunnel (as well as lower cervical spine and brachial plexus) can manifest as primary ulnar hand and wrist complaints (**Fig. 4**).

Grip strength testing using a dynamometer can be useful for several reasons. Grip strength ratios of the injured to noninjured side have been found to correlate with the DASH (disabilities of the arm, shoulder, and hand) score, are quicker to perform, and do not rely on subjective questionnaires.[9] The normal ratio of dominant to nondominant hands in healthy volunteers was found to be

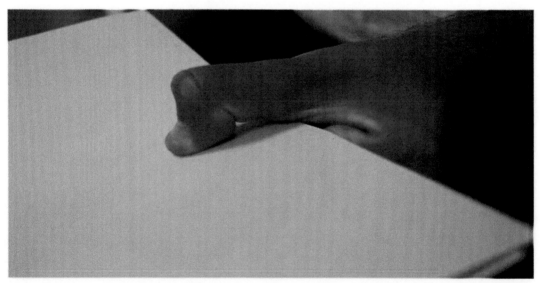

Fig. 3. Key pinch against a piece of paper showing a positive Froment sign (IP flexion) and mild Jeanne sign (metacarpophalangeal hyperextension).

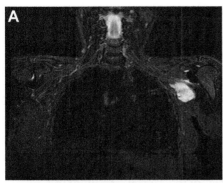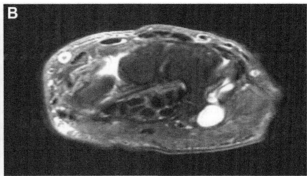

Fig. 4. (*A*) Chest MRI showing a lower brachial plexus tumor that presented with complaints of ulnar-sided hand and wrist pain. (*B*) Axial wrist MRI showing both a hamate hook nonunion and a ganglion within Guyon canal in a patient presenting with ulnar wrist pain.

0.97.[9] Discrepancy beyond that should raise suspicion for injury. It has been proposed that grip strength testing might help clinicians gauge sincerity of effort, especially in instances in which disability may be tied to secondary gain. For instance, disability exaggeration has been reported to confound up to a third of worker's compensation cases.[10] However, although rapid exchange and 5-station grip testing can provide valuable insight, no study to date has established a reliable protocol to predict sincerity of effort.[11]

A vascular examination should begin with observation, looking for any digital ulcerations, splinter hemorrhages, or hand swelling/discoloration (**Fig. 5**). This observation is followed by assessing capillary refill in all digits and palpable pulses at the wrist. Differential perfusion can signify Raynaud phenomenon or disorder of the ulnar artery at Guyon canal. The Allen test verifies that both the ulnar and radial artery are contributing to perfusion of the hand, and is performed by placing the examiner's thumbs over the radial and ulnar artery simultaneously and asking the patient to make a tight fist, effectively exsanguinating the palm. When the patient opens up the hand, the examiner releases pressure from either the ulnar or radial artery alone and assesses whether perfusion to the entire palm is restored. The maneuver is

then repeated for the other artery. Disorder affecting the ulnar artery, such as aneurysm or thrombosis, or a congenital deficit in the anastomoses between the deep and superficial arches, leads to lack of reperfusion when only the ulnar artery is released during Allen test.

A sensory examination should be performed to assess sensory threshold using a Semmes-Weinstein type monofilament, and innervation density with 2-point discrimination. Sensation in the ulnar nerve distribution of the small and ulnar side of the ring finger should be compared with that in the ipsilateral median nerve distribution as well as with the contralateral hand.

The most important aspect of diagnosing ulnar-sided wrist pain is knowledge of the underlying palpable structures of the ulnar wrist to enable the examiner to accurately identify disorder with high specificity. When palpating the patient's wrist, the examiner essentially completes a full circuit of these structures, saving the patient's self-reported point of maximal pain or tenderness for last: premature palpation of the painful structure may confound the rest of the examination, because the patient may feel that everything hurts and be more reluctant to be examined.

The examiner must know the anatomy of the wrist and be able to visualize where the structures

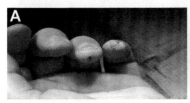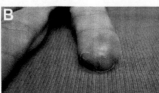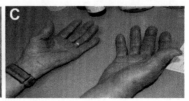

Fig. 5. Various vascular causes of patients presenting with ulnar-sided hand complaints: (*A*) fingertip ulcerations from emboli secondary to hypothenar hammer syndrome; (*B*) small finger ecchymosis from cardiac emboli; (*C*) diffuse hand swelling from a subclavian deep vein thrombosis.

lie under the skin; this is what is meant by surface anatomy. **Fig. 6** shows what examiners should be able to visualize in their "mind's eye" when looking at a patient's hand and wrist. The authors recommend that readers practice palpating the structures described on their own wrists while reading through the following paragraphs.

Start by identifying the pisiform (A4): it is the bony prominence immediately distal to the wrist flexion crease ulnarly. The flexor carpi ulnaris (FCU) (A5) tendon inserts onto the pisiform and is easily palpated moving proximally along the ulnar volar wrist.

Next, place your thumb IP joint directly over the pisiform, aiming toward the ring finger. The tip of your thumb will land over the hook of the hamate, which feels like a subtle and deep bony prominence.

The ulnar head is immediately palpable in the ulnar dorsal quadrant of the wrist and the ulnar styloid is the most dorsal and distal aspect of the ulnar head. Starting on the ulnar styloid, let the tip of your examining finger slide volarly into a groove: this is the fovea (A*), where the TFCC is located. The ECU tendon (A1), which travels within the sixth dorsal compartment in its own separate subsheath, overlies the dorsal ulna and is most easily visualized with the forearm in full supination while abducting the fingers. Its course to its insertion on the base of the fifth metacarpal (A6) is in a straight line with the forearm pronated and oblique with the forearm in supination. Therefore, supination is best for visualizing the tendon and eliciting instability, whereas pronation is the preferred position for immobilization and protection of the ECU. Starting at the fifth metacarpal shaft dorsally, palpate proximally to the fifth CMC joint. Proximal to the joint is the dorsum of the hamate, and radial to the fifth CMC joint is the fourth CMC joint.

Next, palpate the Lister tubercle over the dorsal distal radius. Move 1 cm ulnar along the distal radius until you reach the edge of the radius, into the distal radioulnar joint (DRUJ). From the DRUJ, move directly distal and find a small groove: this is the LT interval.

Having identified a specific anatomic area of tenderness to palpation, the next step is to use specialized maneuvers that have been described to aid in the diagnosis of specific disorders.

Several provocative maneuvers or special tests have been described to diagnose certain common disorders. These maneuvers should be performed

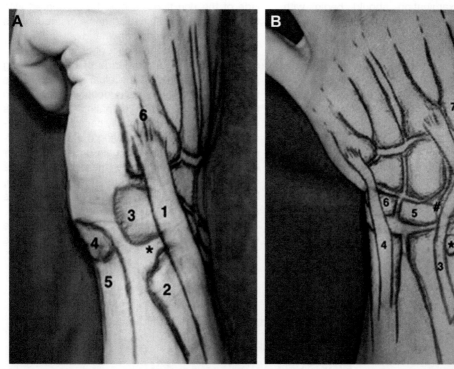

Fig. 6. (A) 1, ECU tendon; 2, ulnar head; 3, triquetrum; 4, pisiform; 5, flexor carpi ulnaris tendon; 6, fifth metacarpal base. Asterisk (*) indicates fovea. (B) 1, Distal radius; 2, extensor carpi radialis brevis/extensor carpi radialis longus; 3, extensor pollicis longus; 4, ECU; 5, lunate; 6, triquetrum; 7, first metacarpal base. Asterisk (*) indicates Lister tubercle; hash (#) indicates scapholunate interval.

to confirm a suspected diagnosis or more confidently rule one out, rather than as a screening tool.

Ulnocarpal Stress Test

The ulnocarpal stress test, described by Nakamura and colleagues[12] as being 100% sensitive for pathology on the ulnar side of the wrist, involves applying axial pressure to the patient's fist with the patient's elbow held in flexion and the wrist in ulnar deviation, and then passively ranging the wrist in pronation and supination. The test was not able to differentiate between several causes of ulnar-sided wrist pain, including TFCC tears, LT tears, DRUJ arthritis, and ulnar impaction syndrome and therefore is not considered specific, but it remains a valuable screening tool for ulnar wrist disorder.[3,12] A variation of the ulnocarpal stress test is the press test, described by Lester and colleagues[13] as being 100% sensitive and highly specific for TFCC tears in patients with the appropriate pretest clinical suspicion. The press test simply involves the patient pushing up from the seated position by gripping the sides of the seat portion of a chair. A positive test is defined as reproducing the pain that prompted clinical evaluation. Although there are methodological limitations, the test is likely to be equivalent to the Nakamura ulnocarpal stress test.

Hook of Hamate Fracture

If pain is elicited with palpation directly over the hook of the hamate, a hook of the hamate fracture or nonunion should be suspected. The hook of hamate pull test was described by Wright and colleagues[5] to aid in the diagnosis of hook of the hamate fractures, which can produce vague pain and remain occult on plain radiographs. The test involves the reproduction of pain with flexion of the fourth and fifth digits against resistance while the wrist is held in ulnar deviation. The hamate hook serves as a pulley for the ulnar digital flexors. The tendons' course around the hook becomes more oblique in ulnar deviation, causing increased pressure on the hook and more pain in the setting of injury. Radially deviating the wrist should lessen the patient's pain.

Pisiform-Triquetrum Arthritis

If a patient has pain with direct palpation of the pisiform in the absence of trauma, pisiform-triquetrum (PT) arthritis should be considered as a diagnosis, especially in the older population. PT arthritis is an easily missed source of ulnar wrist pain and can be a confounder to accurate testing of the LT interval as well given the direct pressure applied to the pisiform during many of these provocative maneuvers. The pisiform tracking test (also known as the PT grind test) is performed with the patient's wrist in slight flexion to relax the FCU tendon. The pisiform is grasped between index and thumb while stabilizing the dorsal aspect of the wrist with the other hand. Pressure is applied onto the pisiform and into the PT joint while "shucking" the pisiform radially and ulnarly. Pain with or without crepitus may be present in patients with disorder at this joint.[2]

Lunotriquetral Ligament Tears

Kleinman[7] has written extensively about the examination of LT tears.[7] Because partial LT tears do not produce findings on radiographs, the physical examination is deemed critical. Kleinman[7] describes 3 possible maneuvers: a ballottment test, a shuck test, and his own shear test, which he indicates is more sensitive and specific than the previous 2.[7] Pain and/or increased laxity compared with the opposite side is considered positive for all of these tests.

In the ballottment test, attributed to Linscheid, the examiner places a thumb on the ulnar or medial aspect of the patient's pisiform and applies pressure radially while stabilizing the rest of the patient's wrist and forearm. Kleinman[7] warns that this test lacks specificity, because it simultaneously stresses other structures, including the ulnocarpal ligaments, the TFCC, and extrinsic radiocarpal ligaments. In the shuck test, attributed to Reagan, the triquetrum and pisiform are grasped as a unit between the examiner's index and thumb, and shucked in the dorsal to palmar direction, exerting stress at the LT joint.

For Kleinman shear test, the examiner places a thumb over the patient's pisiform and the other thumb over the dorsal lunate while stabilizing the forearm with interlaced hands. The advantage of this test according to its author is that very gradual pressure can be applied, resulting in incremental shear forces across the LT joint. However, because the loading of the triquetrum passes through the PT joint, it is important to rule out PT arthritis using the pisiform tracking test described earlier for these maneuvers. Additional causes that may result in false-positive findings during LT provocative testing include avascular necrosis of the lunate (Kienbock disease), FCU tendonitis, proximal hamate arthrosis, or a triquetral avulsion fracture.

DISTAL RADIOULNAR JOINT ARTHRITIS AND INSTABILITY

Pain caused by DRUJ arthritis can be reproduced by the DRUJ compression test, in which the distal radius and ulna are compressed against each. Both bones should be gripped 1 to 2 cm proximal to the ulnar head and a compressive load applied. To test for DRUJ instability, which may be distinct from pain, the piano key or DRUJ ballotment test is simply the process of shucking the distal ulna or ulnar head from volar to dorsal against a fixed radius stabilized by the other hand.[14] This maneuver should be performed in pronation, neutral, and supination, because the ligaments stabilizing the DRUJ in pronation and supination are distinct, and compared with the contralateral side (Video 1).[3]

Extensor Carpi Ulnaris Subsheath

The spectrum of ECU disorder, from tendonitis to subluxation and dislocation, can be reproduced by the synergy test, described by Ruland and colleagues.[15] The test is helpful in differentiating ECU disorder from TFCC disorder, which can be a diagnostic challenge at times given the close proximity of the structures and similar subjective complaints. First, the patient is asked to fully supinate the wrist (resulting in a more oblique path of the ECU to its insertion). Next, the patient abducts the thumb and long finger against resistance, which synergistically fires the ECU. Sharp pain with this maneuver supports a diagnosis of ECU tendonitis. If there is a tear of the ECU subsheath, the tendon may visibly subluxate, or even frankly dislocate. Subluxation and dislocation can also be reproduced with the ice cream scoop motion, which involves having the patient perform flexion, ulnar deviation, and supination of the wrist actively and observing for signs of ECU instability (Video 2).

Triangular Fibrocartilage Complex

In addition, the TFCC is often considered to be one of the most complex and confusing structures of the ulnar side of the wrist. Specific provocative testing of distinct structural components of the TFCC have been described.[16] Tenderness to palpation at the ulnar fovea alone has been shown to be both sensitive (95.2%) and specific (86.5%) for TFCC disorder (either a tear of the deep fibers, also called ligamentum subcruentum, or of the ulnotriquetral ligament).[17]

Provocative testing of the TFCC relies on an understanding of the TFCC's function and anatomy. The TFCC serves 2 functions via 2 distinct anatomic structures. First, it diffuses load transmission to the ulna via a central cartilaginous disc. Second, the peripheral fibers of the TFCC stabilize and guide the rotation of the DRUJ in a controlled fashion despite the noncongruent articular surfaces of the ulnar head and styloid notch.

Kleinman[16] emphasizes the importance of the physical examination to assess the deep fibers of the TFCC (also known as the ligamentum subcruentum or deep radial and ulnar ligaments) because they cannot be visualized arthroscopically through standard radiocarpal portals.

The dorsal and volar deep fibers are tested sequentially by placing each on maximum tension. To assess the deep dorsal TFCC, the patient's wrist is placed in full supination and the examiner applies a palmarly directed force to the distal ulna. In contrast, the deep volar TFCC fibers are tested by placing the patient's wrist in full pronation and applying a dorsally directed force to the ulnar head while assessing pain and or instability compared with the contralateral side. An easy way to remember which fibers are being tested is to notice that the aspect of the patient's hand that is visible to the examiner corresponds to the fibers being tested: in supination, the examiner sees the dorsum of the patient's hand, meaning the deep dorsal fibers are being tested.

At this point in the encounter, the clinician should have narrowed the differential diagnosis down to only a few possibilities based on the history and the physical examination. For instance, if a young patient has maximal tenderness to palpation over the pisiform after a recent fall onto the outstretched hand, a fracture or contusion of the pisiform is likely. However, if the same area is tender but the onset of symptoms was insidious in a young and active patient, FCU insertional tendonitis is more likely. In older patients without recent trauma, PT arthritis is a common disorder.

Injections of local anesthetic with or without steroid in the office can serve both diagnostic and therapeutic purposes. If ambiguity remains between multiple diagnoses, injection of a small amount of anesthetic into a specific location is an efficient and cost-effective tool. For injection into specific joints, such as either the PT, LT, or fourth or fifth MP joints, the use of an office mini C-arm or ultrasonography to confirm needle position may be helpful. An injection may also be performed in a tendon subsheath such as the ECU. In patients with isolated extra-articular disorder involving the ECU, such an injection would be expected to alleviate their symptoms, and the addition of corticosteroid constitutes the first-line and possibly definitive treatment[15] For intra-articular disorder, an injection may be performed into the DRUJ or around the TFCC.

In summary, although the ulnar side of the wrist is anatomically intricate, and pain in this area can be caused by a wide array of disorders, a systematic approach to the history and physical examination often allows knowledgeable clinicians to reach a diagnosis in the office. Understanding the surface anatomy is critical, and developing confidence in palpating the structures of the ulnar side of the wrist to establish the point of maximal tenderness is a keystone of diagnosis.

CLINICS CARE POINTS

- The History and Physical Examination are critical to determining the etiology and guiding treatment of ulnar sided wrist pain.
- Familiarity with the surface anatomy of the ulnar side of the wrist allows for high levels of diagnostic accuracy in the office.
- The point of maximal tenderness to palpation along with specific provocative maneuvers often yield a diagnosis.
- Differential injections in the office, in particular intra-articular vs. ECU subsheath injections can have both diagnostic and therapeutic value.
- A robust differential diagnosis based on the History and Physical should be established prior to obtaining advanced imaging which has a high rate of incidental findings, especially in older patients.

SUPPLEMENTARY DATA

Supplementary data related to this article can be found online at https://doi.org/10.1016/j.hcl.2021. 06.002.

DISCLOSURE

The authors have no relevant commercial or financial disclosures and received no funding for this work.

REFERENCES

1. Diaz RI. Ulnar-Sided Wrist Pain: A Master Skills Publication. J Hand Surg Am 2014. https://doi.org/10.1016/j.jhsa.2013.11.005.

2. Shin AY, Deitch MA, Sachar K, et al. Ulnar-sided wrist pain: diagnosis and treatment. Instr Course Lect 2005;54:115–28.

3. Sachar K. Ulnar-sided wrist pain: Evaluation and treatment of triangular fibrocartilage complex tears, ulnocarpal impaction syndrome, and lunotriquetral ligament tears. J Hand Surg Am 2012. https://doi.org/10.1016/j.jhsa.2012.04.036.

4. Dasilva MF, Goodman AD, Gil JA, et al. Evaluation of ulnar-sided wrist pain. J Am Acad Orthop Surg 2017. https://doi.org/10.5435/JAAOS-D-16-00407.

5. Wright TW, Moser MW, Sahajpal DT. Hook of hamate pull test. J Hand Surg Am 2010. https://doi.org/10.1016/j.jhsa.2010.08.024.

6. Montalvan B, Parier J, Brasseur JL, et al. Extensor carpi ulnaris injuries in tennis players: A study of 28 cases. Br J Sports Med 2006. https://doi.org/10.1136/bjsm.2005.023275.

7. Kleinman WB. Physical examination of the wrist: Useful provocative maneuvers. J Hand Surg Am 2015. https://doi.org/10.1016/j.jhsa.2015.01.016.

8. Wagstaff S, Smith OV, Wood PHN. Verbal pain descriptors used by patients with arthritis. Ann Rheum Dis 1985. https://doi.org/10.1136/ard.44.4.262.

9. Beumer A, Lindau TR. Grip strength ratio: A grip strength measurement that correlates well with DASH score in different hand/wrist conditions. BMC Musculoskelet Disord 2014. https://doi.org/10.1186/1471-2474-15-336.

10. Mittenberg W, Patton C, Canyock EM, et al. Base rates of malingering and symptom exaggeration. J Clin Exp Neuropsychol 2002. https://doi.org/10.1076/jcen.24.8.1094.8379.

11. Sindhu BS, Shechtman O, Veazie PJ. Identifying sincerity of effort based on the combined predictive ability of multiple grip strength tests. J Hand Ther 2012. https://doi.org/10.1016/j.jht.2012.03.007.

12. Nakamura R, Horii E, Imaeda T, et al. The ulnocarpal stress test in the diagnosis of ulnar-sided wrist pain. J Hand Surg Eur Vol 1997. https://doi.org/10.1016/S0266-7681(97)80432-9.

13. Lester B, Halbrecht J, Levy IM, et al. "Press test" for office diagnosis of triangular fibrocartilage complex tears of the wrist. Ann Plast Surg 1995. https://doi.org/10.1097/00000637-199507000-00009.

14. Szabo RM. Distal radioulnar joint instability. Instr Course Lect 2007;36(5):305–13.

15. Ruland RT, Hogan CJ. The ECU Synergy Test: An Aid to Diagnose ECU Tendonitis. J Hand Surg Am 2008. https://doi.org/10.1016/j.jhsa.2008.08.018.

16. Kleinman WB. Stability of the distal radioulnar joint. Fractures and injuries of the distal radius and carpus. The Cutting Edge, Philadelphia (PA), 2009. p. 261-274.

17. Tay SC, Tomita K, Berger RA. The "Ulnar Fovea Sign" for Defining Ulnar Wrist Pain: An Analysis of Sensitivity and Specificity. J Hand Surg Am 2007. https://doi.org/10.1016/j.jhsa.2007.01.022.

Advanced Imaging of Ulnar Wrist Pain

R. Timothy Kreulen, MD[a],*, Suresh K. Nayar, MD[a], Yasmin Alfaki[b], Dawn LaPorte, MD[a], Shadpour Demehri, MD[c]

KEYWORDS

• Ulna • Wrist • Imaging • Advanced

KEY POINTS

- Ulnar wrist anatomy is intricate and complex.
- Broadly, the differential diagnosis for ulnar wrist pathologic condition can be broken down into 5 categories: fracture, neurovascular pathologic condition, osseous abnormalities, tendinopathies, and ligamentous injuries.
- Current advanced imaging modalities include ultrasound, computed tomography, and MRI.
- A strong understanding of the anatomy, differential diagnosis, and advanced imaging modalities is crucial for proper treatment of patients with ulnar wrist pain.

INTRODUCTION

The cause of ulnar-sided wrist pain can be a diagnostic challenge when relying purely on clinical examination.[1] The ulnar-sided wrist is composed of complex and delicate osseous and soft tissue structures. Osseous components include the distal ulna and proximal carpal bones, including the lunate, triquetrum, and pisiform. Soft tissue components include the ulnocarpal and radioulnar ligaments; extensor carpi ulnaris (ECU) and flexor carpi ulnaris (FCU) tendons; ulnar artery and nerve; and the triangular fibrocartilage complex (TFCC). Structural damage to any of these components can result in pain and instability. The proximity of these structures makes it difficult to determine the exact source of pain.[2] Furthermore, age-related degenerative but asymptomatic changes, such as TFCC tears, may have overlapping imaging features with symptomatic pathologic condition.[3]

Ulnar-sided wrist pain can be acute or chronic. Fractures, ulnar artery thrombosis and aneurysm, tendon ruptures, or ligamentous injury can result in acute pain. Other injuries, such as ulnar nerve compression in Guyon canal; osseous abnormalities (ie, Madelung deformity); distal radioulnar joint (DRUJ) and pisotriquetral arthritis; tendon subluxation, dislocation, or tendonitis; chronic TFCC tear; and ulnar abutment syndrome, can lead to chronic pain.

To successfully diagnose and optimally care for patients with ulnar-sided wrist pain, radiologists and orthopedic surgeons must have a thorough understanding of the anatomy and roles that ultrasound (US), computed tomography (CT), and MRI play in diagnosis. In this review, the authors provide a focused overview of ulnar wrist anatomy with particular emphasis on the optimal imaging modality for each anatomic component. They then present differential diagnoses categorized by the type of injury. Finally, the authors examine indications for different advanced imaging modalities, including US, CT, and MRI.

NORMAL ANATOMY

The distal ulna articulates with the lunate, triquetrum, and pisiform. Distally, the hamate articulates

---

The authors declare no relevant financial disclosures.
^a Johns Hopkins Department of Orthopaedic Surgery, 601 North Caroline Street 5th Floor, Baltimore, MD 21205, USA; ^b Johns Hopkins University, 3400 North Charles Street, Mason Hall, Baltimore, MD 21218, USA; ^c Johns Hopkins Department of Musculoskeletal Radiology, 601 North Caroline Street 5th Floor, Baltimore, MD 21205, USA
* Corresponding author.
E-mail address: rkreule1@jhmi.edu

Hand Clin 37 (2021) 477–486
https://doi.org/10.1016/j.hcl.2021.06.012

with the triquetrum and small and ring finger metacarpals. The distal ulna also articulates with the radius to form the DRUJ. Twenty percent of DRUJ stability is provided by the sigmoid notch, a bony articulation between the distal radius and ulnar head.[4] There can be a large degree of variability in ulnar variance, which is defined as the relative alignment between the distal ulna and ulnar-side of the distal radius[5] (**Fig. 1**). Positive ulnar variance is defined as projection of the ulna beyond the distal edge of the radius by more than 1 mm. It may increase joint contact pressure between the distal ulna and proximal carpal row, leading to ulnar abutment syndrome and subsequent arthritis. In contrast, negative ulnar variance is defined as ulnar height ≤1 to 2 mm shorter than the distal radius. It can be associated with Kienbock disease, whereby the distal ulna is offloaded, and more force is transmitted through the lunate. In general, osseous structures are optimally

evaluated using high-resolution CT. MRI can have added value in detection of osseous compositional abnormalities, such as osteonecrosis or bone marrow edema, in the setting of trauma.

The primary ligamentous structures include the ulnocarpal, radioulnar, and lunotriquetral ligaments. Injury of the ulnocarpal ligaments can result in supination of the carpus.[6] The radioulnar ligaments stabilize the wrist during pronation-supination motion[7] and protect against both dorsal and palmar translation of the DRUJ.[4] Ligamentous structures are best seen and evaluated on MRI.

The ulnar wrist tendons are the FCU and ECU. In addition to flexion, extension, and ulnar-deviation of the wrist, they act as dynamic stabilizers.[8] They are best seen on MRI, but US is gaining popularity, as it allows for dynamic evaluation.

The ulnar artery and nerve make up the ulnar neurovascular bundle. At the level of the wrist, the ulnar nerve is composed of both motor and sensory branches. The ulnar artery terminates into the superficial palmar arch, which anastomoses with branches from the radial artery. The neurovascular bundle can be evaluated on US, MRI, and CT.

The TFCC is perhaps the most complex structure to evaluate in the ulnar wrist. It consists of an articular disc, the ECU tendon subsheath, and radioulnar ligaments. The main functions of the TFCC are to stabilize the DRUJ and act as a shock absorber between the ulna and carpus.[9] Imaging may reveal both acute and chronic tears. These tears present a challenge to both diagnose and treat because of the TFCC's tenuous blood supply. Although the peripheral 15% to 20% is well vascularized, its central portion is avascular.[10] In addition, the percentage of asymptomatic TFCC tears increases with age. This is a distinct pathologic condition from posttraumatic TFCC tears.

DIFFERENTIAL DIAGNOSIS

The differential diagnosis for ulnar-sided wrist pain is broad. The breadth of pathologic conditions makes the diagnosis and treatment of ulnar-sided wrist pain challenging. In general, there are 5 categories of ulnar wrist pain pathologic conditions: fracture, neurovascular pathologic condition, osseous abnormalities, tendinopathies, and ligamentous injuries. Trauma to the ulnar styloid, hamate, pisiform, and fifth metacarpal base should first be evaluated with plain radiography, including standard posteroanterior (PA), lateral, and oblique views. The hook of the hamate fractures may best be appreciated on a carpal tunnel view. Occasionally, a high-resolution CT scan

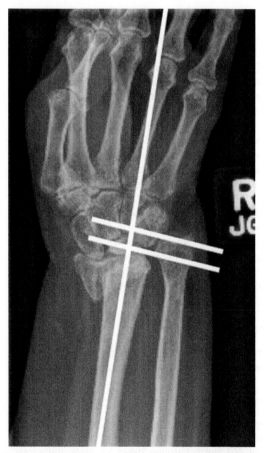

Fig. 1. Anteroposterior radiograph of the right wrist. There is increased ulnar height secondary to shortening of the radius secondary to a displaced, intraarticular comminuted fracture. This is consistent with posttraumatic positive ulnar variance.

can identify an occult injury or better characterize injury patterns for higher-energy trauma.

Neurovascular pathologic conditions include ulnar nerve compression in Guyon canal; ulnar artery thrombosis, aneurysm, pseudoaneurysm; and hypothenar hammer syndrome. US, CT, and MRI are all useful in the setting of neurovascular pathologic condition. The addition of intravenous contrast for CT and MRI can better characterize any discontinuity of the ulnar artery and should be recommended at the clinician and radiologist's discretion.

Osseous abnormalities include Madelung deformity, Kienbock disease, DRUJ arthritis, pisotriquetral arthritis, triquetral avulsion fracture, and impaction syndromes. Most osseous abnormalities can be seen on radiograph. Live fluoroscopy can be used to visualize ulnar abutment. MRI and CT can be useful in gauging bone integrity in avascular pathologic conditions, such as Kienbock.

Tendinopathies may include ECU, FCU, and EDM tendonitis, subluxation, dislocation, or rupture. They are best visualized on US or MRI without contrast.

Finally, ligamentous injuries include TFCC injury, DRUJ instability, midcarpal instability, and lunotriquetral dissociation. These pathologic conditions are best seen on MRI.

ULTRASOUND

US has gained popularity in musculoskeletal radiology because of lack of radiation, low cost, and ability to obtain dynamic images. Its primary utility is in the evaluation of soft tissue, rather than bone.[11] It helps to identify foreign bodies, masses, effusions, tendonitis, compressive neuropathies, and vascular flow.[12,13] US utility is largely operator-dependent, and therefore, its diagnostic performance depends on the examiners' experience.

US can accurately assess FCU and ECU tendons tears and instability (**Fig. 2**). The tendons' paths can be easily tracked. Any discontinuity can represent a tear.[14,15] It can also be used to evaluate the DRUJ. In a cadaveric model, US showed moderate to strong correlation with magnetic resonance arthrography (MRA) for tear diagnosis.[16]

The neurovascular bundle can also be visualized with US. Doppler US can provide detailed information on arterial flow and the presence of vascularity in palpable wrist masses.[17] US can also identify masses or anatomic abnormalities next to the neurovascular bundle contributing to a compressive pathologic condition, such as a ganglion cyst.

US is a dynamic study, which can be useful, especially when evaluating mobile structures. It

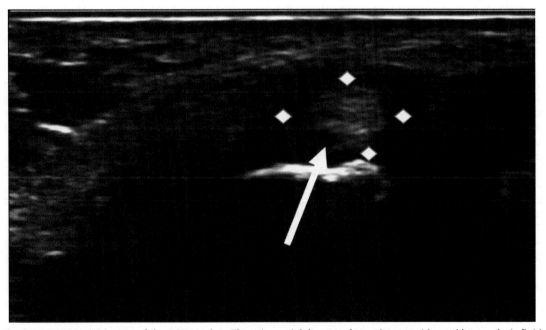

Fig. 2. Transverse US image of the ECU tendon. There is partial, low-grade tearing as evidenced by anechoic fluid within the substance of the tendon (*arrow*). There is also tenosynovitis as evidenced by presence of fluid surrounding the ECU tendon (*diamonds*).

is efficacious in evaluating gliding, anatomic alignment, subluxation, dislocation, and tears of the ECU and FCU tendons.[18–20] However, the dynamic nature of the study may lead to variability in study quality. Therefore, extremity positioning at the time of the study must be considered. For example, the ECU tendon can be displaced 50% volarly when the wrist is positioned in supination, ulnar deviation, and flexion.[19,21]

There are several limitations of US. It is highly user-dependent and has limited application in evaluating osseous anatomy.[11] As with all imaging studies, its results must be correlated with the patient's clinical examination. High false positive rates have been reported. For example, in 1 study of 26 asymptomatic tennis players, US demonstrated ECU tendinopathy in 92% and instability in 73% of subjects.[22]

COMPUTED TOMOGRAPHY

CT scan is a common and versatile imaging modality. Its relative speed and wide availability have led to wider adoption in evaluating wrist injuries. One of its major indications is evaluating osseous anatomy. CT also allows for rapid 2-dimensional (2D) and 3-dimensional (3D) imaging,[23] which can be valuable in evaluating anatomic or injury patterns difficult to discern on plain radiography.[2,24,25] For example, CT can easily evaluate the hook of hamate morphology leading to improved fracture detection and may be particularly useful in nondisplaced fractures.[26] CT technology is evolving. Cone-beam CT may outperform conventional multidirectional CT in detecting carpal fractures.[27]

CT can be combined with arthrography to provide precise imaging of ligamentous and osseous structures.[28] CT arthrography is best done when contrast is injected following established protocols and combined with multiplanar reformats.[29] These protocols have been developed for many anatomic structures, such as the TFCC.[30] Literature shows that CT arthrography outperforms conventional arthrography when evaluating wrist interosseous ligaments and the TFCC.[31] There is also evidence that it is equivalent to MRA for TFCC pathologic condition.[32] Compared with wrist arthroscopy, CT arthrography has high sensitivity (88%–91%) and specificity (85%–95%) for central TFCC tears. In peripheral TFCC tears, specificity is high (94%–97%), but sensitivity is low (30%–40%).[28]

Four-dimensional CT (4D-CT) is a remarkable and novel CT advancement in the evaluation of dynamic abnormalities of small peripheral joints, such as the knee, ankle, and wrist.[33–35] In this modality, multiple traditional 3D-CT scans are obtained as the extremity is ranged. The 2D and 3D images can be combined to allow for dynamic structural evaluation.[36] The technique is validated for analyzing dynamic abnormalities during various wrist motions[37] and can be used to quantify joint instability.[38] Pathologic conditions in which 4D-CT has shown utility include carpal instability owing to intrinsic (eg, scapholunate interosseous ligaments) and extrinsic ligament injuries (Fig. 3), DRUJ instability, and ulnar impaction syndrome.[39–42] It can also help diagnose rare entities that can be difficult to discern on physical examination, radiographs, and conventional CT, or MRI examinations. For example, it has been used in the diagnosis of pisotriquetral instability.[39] Despite the promising applications of 4D-CT, it is important to note that before motion of structures can be deemed pathologic, normal values must be established using asymptomatic wrist examinations.[40,41]

Finally, the addition of contrast can be used to evaluate ulnar artery patency. This may be helpful for acute trauma or to characterize chronic vascular diseases, such as thromboangiitis obliterans, which may involve ulnar-sided vasculature.

MRI

MRI is a versatile imaging modality with tremendous utility in the detailed assessment of both osseous and soft tissue pathologic condition. It is crucial to obtain thin sections with a high spatial resolution to ensure optimal evaluation of small wrist structures.[43] Therefore, a high-resolution MRI is needed.[44] To obtain high-resolution images, a powerful magnet is used. A 3.0-T MRI has been shown to outperform a 1.5-T MRI when evaluating wrist ligaments (Fig. 4) and the TFCC.[45] Therefore, 3.0-T MRI is currently the standard-of-care MRI modality for ulnar-sided wrist pain.[46]

Like all imaging modalities, the position of the wrist affects MRI. Therefore, a standardized patient positioning protocol has been established. The standardized position is prone with the hand over the head and a neutral wrist.

Within the ulnar wrist, MRI has been extensively studied regarding its ability to detect TFCC tears (Fig. 5). The evidence regarding its efficacy is mixed. In 1 study, it was shown to have a sensitivity of 100%, a specificity of 90%, and an accuracy of 97% for tear detection. With regards to the location of the tear, MRI had a sensitivity of 100%, a specificity of 75%, and an accuracy of 92%.[47] However, another study has shown lower efficacy with sensitivity and specificity as low as

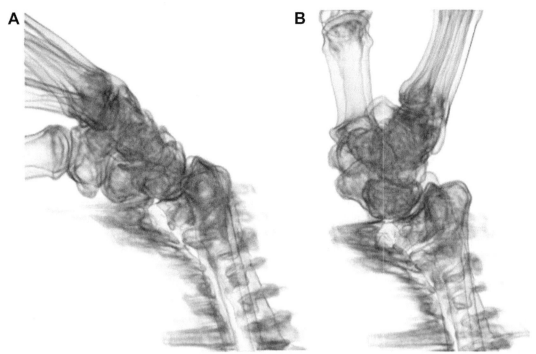

Fig. 3. 4D-CT scan of a patient with persistent ulnar-sided wrist pain and clicking following open reduction and internal fixation of a distal radius fracture. The images show dynamic subluxation of the lunate at the radiocarpal joint as the wrist is brought from flexion (*A*) into extension (*B*), which corresponds to clicking during the flexion-extension motion.

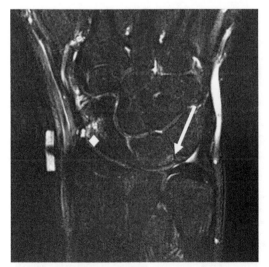

Fig. 4. Fat-saturated T2-weighted coronal MRI of the wrist in a patient with ulnar-sided wrist pain. There is a low-grade, partial-thickness tear of the lunotri-quetral ligament with edema of the adjacent lunate (*arrow*). An additional finding is an osseous contusion of the scaphoid fracture (*diamond*).

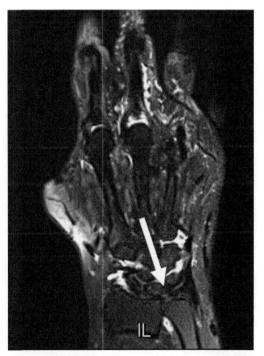

Fig. 5. MRI coronal (*A*) T1- and (*B*) T2-weighted images demonstrating a lunotriquetral coalition with presumable edema within the coalition site (*arrow*). This is negatively impacted by suboptimal fat saturation (*diamond*).

73% to 76% and 41% to 44%, respectively, for detecting a tear.[48] It must be noted that a high number of asymptomatic wrists will have TFCC pathologic condition on MRI, which has been reported as high as 37.9%,[49] and therefore, reiterates the importance of correlating clinical examination with imaging findings.

Although CT is the mainstay for fracture detection, MRI is also accurate in detection of subtle osseous injuries in patients with posttraumatic ulnar-sided wrist pain. The fracture is highlighted by bone marrow edema, detectable on T2 sequences. However, there is a potential for false positives representing purely trabecular fractures or bone bruises.[50] Other osseous abnormalities, such as coalitions, may be noted (**Fig. 6**).

Another main indication for MRI is evaluating tendinopathy (**Fig. 7**). One study showed a 57% sensitivity and 88% specificity in evaluating ECU pathologic condition. It should be reiterated that ECU position and dynamics are dependent on pronosupination of the wrist. Therefore, images can be obtained in both protonation and supination to best define the anatomy.[51] As previously mentioned, MRI is valuable in evaluating for tendon rupture.[52] Tear characteristics can be accurately quantified. For example, MRI has

been shown to be effective at differentiating complete from partial tears.[53] However, MRI may also overdiagnose interstitial tendon tearing, as patches of linear signal may correspond to separate slips within a tendon and not an actual tear.

Kienbock disease, or avascular necrosis of the lunate, is also best evaluated on MRI. MRI can allow for early detection. Early disease is characterized by low signal intensity on T1.[2] MRI may also show lunate vascular patterns, which are more prone to Kienbock.

Ulnar impaction syndrome is caused by repetitive microtrauma from the ulna impacting the carpus. It is associated with ulnar positivity. A focal radial-sided lesion of the ulnar head may correspond to an ulnar-sided lesion of the lunate.[54] Soft tissue enhancement just distal to the ulnar styloid process may be seen as well.

MRI can be supplemented with contrast. Direct and indirect MRA can be used. Direct MRA involves contrast injected directly into the joint. The intraarticular contrast allows for improved visualization of anatomic structures. It also distends the joint, which may help in anatomic differentiation.[55] This makes it a useful study to evaluate wrist ligaments and the TFCC. A meta-analysis showed direct MRA to be superior to conventional

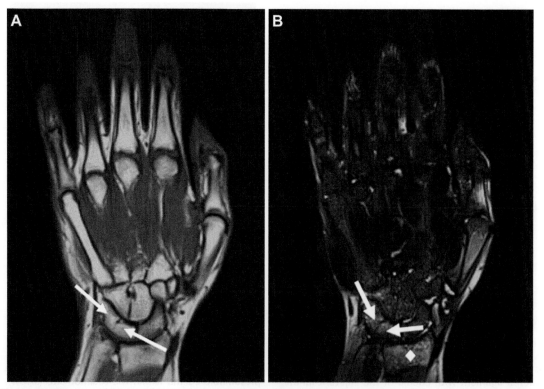

Fig. 6. T2 MRI coronal image of the wrist in a patient with a history of atraumatic ulnar wrist pain. The image showcases a central TFCC perforation (*arrows*), likely secondary to degeneration.

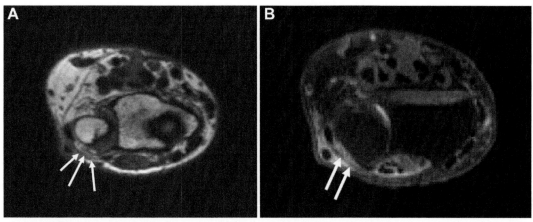

Fig. 7. Axial MRI T1- (*A*) and (*B*) T2-weighted images demonstrating subluxation of the ECU with tearing of the extensor retinaculum (*arrows*).

MRI in detecting TFCC pathologic condition. MRA had a sensitivity and specificity of 84% and 85%, compared with 75% and 81%, respectively, for conventional MRI. However, direct MRA has some disadvantages. It can be expensive and invasive because contrast has to be directed directly into the joint.[56] It has mostly been replaced by indirect MRI given its high false negative rates, pain with the contrast injection, and risk of chemical synovitis.[2]

Indirect MRA uses intravenous contrast and works through passive joint diffusion. Movement may increase blood flow to the wrist and lead to increased contrast perforation.[57] Early evidence suggested that indirect MRA was excellent for TFCC pathologic condition.[57] However, other literature has shown it to be no better than nonenhanced MRI.[58]

Although MRI is perhaps the most utilitarian imaging modality for the ulnar wrist, it does have limitations. It can be prone to technical factors, which make the studies difficult to interpret.[59] Findings must also be paired with clinical examination. One study showed that the asymptomatic tennis player had an average of 2.64 abnormalities noted on MRIs.[60]

SPECIAL RADIOGRAPHIC VIEWS

Although a detailed discussion of radiographs is outside of the scope of this review, there are several key principles worth mentioning. Standard hand radiographs should be obtained with the shoulder abducted and the elbow flexed at 90°. The PA view should show the ECU tendon groove at the level of or radial to the base of the ulnar styloid.[61] Any rotation can interfere with properly measured ulnar variance. On the lateral view, the pisiform's volar cortex should overlap the middle third of the space between the palmar cortices of the distal scaphoid pole and the head of the capitate.[62]

Specific radiographic views can be obtained to further assess potential pathologic condition. A carpal tunnel view involves extending the wrist and aiming the radiograph beam directly down the proximal carpal row. This view is particularly useful when looking for hook of hamate and pisotriquetral pathologic condition.[63]

Although radiographs discern primarily osseous pathologic condition, certain fracture patterns may be associated with ligamentous injury. For example, ulnar styloid fractures with more than 2 to 4 mm of displacement are associated with TFCC tears and DRUJ instability.[64,65]

SUMMARY

Ulnar wrist pain is a complicated problem with a variety of potential causes, including fracture, neurovascular pathologic condition, osseous abnormalities, tendinopathies, and ligamentous problems. Advanced imaging, including US, CT, and MRI, can be important to aid diagnosis and treatment, and each modality has its own strengths and weaknesses.

CLINICS CARE POINTS

- The differential diagnosis for ulnar wrist pain includes fracture, neurovascular pathologic condition, osseous abnormalities, tendinopathies, and ligamentous injuries.

- Ultrasound provides dynamic images, although it is limited by operator dependence.
- Computed tomography renders excellent evaluation of bony anatomy, and the emergence of 4D computed tomography gives clinicians dynamic information.
- 3.0-T MRI provides valuable diagnostic information for both osseous and soft tissue structures.

REFERENCES

1. Coggins CA. Imaging of ulnar-sided wrist pain. Clin Sports Med 2006;25(3):505–26, vii.
2. Watanabe A, Souza F, Vezeridis PS, et al. Ulnar-sided wrist pain. II. Clinical imaging and treatment. Skeletal Radiol 2010;39(9):837–57.
3. Porteous R, Harish S, Parasu N. Imaging of ulnar-sided wrist pain. Can Assoc Radiol J 2012;63(1): 18–29.
4. Stuart PR, Berger RA, Linscheid RL, et al. The dorsopalmar stability of the distal radioulnar joint. J Hand Surg Am 2000;25(4):689–99.
5. Sachar K. Ulnar-sided wrist pain: evaluation and treatment of triangular fibrocartilage complex tears, ulnocarpal impaction syndrome, and lunotriquetral ligament tears. J Hand Surg Am 2008;33(9):1669–79.
6. Brogan DM, Berger RA, Kakar S. Ulnar-sided wrist pain: a critical analysis review. JBJS Rev 2019; 7(5):e1.
7. Huang JI, Hanel DP. Anatomy and biomechanics of the distal radioulnar joint. Hand Clin 2012;28(2):157–63.
8. Esplugas M, Garcia-Elias M, Lluch A, et al. Role of muscles in the stabilization of ligament-deficient wrists. J Hand Ther 2016;29(2):166–74.
9. Sasao S, Beppu M, Kihara H, et al. An anatomical study of the ligaments of the ulnar compartment of the wrist. Hand Surg 2003;8(2):219–26.
10. Thiru RG, Ferlic DC, Clayton ML, et al. Arterial anatomy of the triangular fibrocartilage of the wrist and its surgical significance. J Hand Surg Am 1986; 11(2):258–63.
11. Heuck A, Bonél H, Stäbler A, et al. Imaging in sports medicine: hand and wrist. Eur J Radiol 1997;26(1): 2–15.
12. Read JW, Conolly WB, Lanzetta M, et al. Diagnostic ultrasound of the hand and wrist. J Hand Surg Am 1996;21(6):1004–10.
13. Starr HM, Sedgley MD, Means KR, et al. Ultrasonography for hand and wrist conditions. J Am Acad Orthop Surg 2016;24(8):544–54.
14. Fornage BD, Rifkin MD. Ultrasound examination of the hand and foot. Radiol Clin North Am 1988; 26(1):109–29.
15. Bianchi S, Martinoli C, Abdelwahab IF. High-frequency ultrasound examination of the wrist and hand. Skeletal Radiol 1999;28(3):121–9.
16. Buck FM, Nico MAC, Gheno R, et al. Ultrasonographic evaluation of degenerative changes in the distal radioulnar joint: correlation of findings with gross anatomy and MR arthrography in cadavers. Eur J Radiol 2011;77(2):215–21.
17. Olchowy C, Soliński D, Łasecki M, et al. Wrist ultrasound examination - scanning technique and ultrasound anatomy. Part 2: ventral wrist. J Ultrason 2017;17(69):123–8.
18. Smith J, Finnoff JT. Diagnostic and interventional musculoskeletal ultrasound: part 2. Clinical applications. PM R 2009;1(2):162–77.
19. Pratt RK, Hoy GA, Bass Franzcr C. Extensor carpi ulnaris subluxation or dislocation? Ultrasound measurement of tendon excursion and normal values. Hand Surg 2004;9(2):137–43.
20. Khoury V, Cardinal E, Bureau NJ. Musculoskeletal sonography: a dynamic tool for usual and unusual disorders. AJR Am J Roentgenol 2007;188(1):W63–73.
21. Lee KS, Ablove RH, Singh S, et al. Ultrasound imaging of normal displacement of the extensor carpi ulnaris tendon within the ulnar groove in 12 forearm-wrist positions. AJR Am J Roentgenol 2009;193(3):651–5.
22. Sole JS, Wisniewski SJ, Newcomer KL, et al. Sonographic evaluation of the extensor carpi ulnaris in asymptomatic tennis players. PM R 2015;7(3): 255–63.
23. Kaewlai R, Avery LL, Asrani AV, et al. Multidetector CT of carpal injuries: anatomy, fractures, and fracture-dislocations. Radiographics 2008;28(6): 1771–84.
24. Imaging of hamate bone fractures in conventional X-rays and high-resolution computed tomography. An in vitro study - PubMed. Available at: https://pubmed.ncbi.nlm.nih.gov/9888053/. Accessed May 7, 2020.
25. Etli I, Kozaci N, Avci M, et al. Comparison of the diagnostic accuracy of X-ray and computed tomography in patients with wrist injury. Injury 2020;51(3): 651–5.
26. Imaging recognition of morphological variants at the midcarpal joint - PubMed. Available at: https://pubmed-ncbi-nlm-nih-gov.proxy1.library.jhu.edu/19497684/. Accessed August 17, 2020.
27. Gibney B, Smith M, Moughty A, et al. Incorporating cone-beam CT into the diagnostic algorithm for suspected radiocarpal fractures: a new standard of care? AJR Am J Roentgenol 2019;213(5):1117–23.
28. Bille B, Harley B, Cohen H. A comparison of CT arthrography of the wrist to findings during wrist arthroscopy. J Hand Surg 2007;32(6):834–41.
29. Moser T, Dosch J-C, Moussaoui A, et al. Multidetector CT arthrography of the wrist joint: how to do it. Radiographics 2008;28(3):787–800 [quiz 911].

30. Moritomo H, Arimitsu S, Kubo N, et al. Computed tomography arthrography using a radial plane view for the detection of triangular fibrocartilage complex foveal tears. J Hand Surg Am 2015;40(2):245–51.

31. Theumann N, Favarger N, Schnyder P, et al. Wrist ligament injuries: value of post-arthrography computed tomography. Skeletal Radiol 2001;30(2):88–93.

32. Omlor G, Jung M, Grieser T, et al. Depiction of the triangular fibro-cartilage in patients with ulnar-sided wrist pain: comparison of direct multi-slice CT arthrography and direct MR arthrography. Eur Radiol 2009;19(1):147–51.

33. Demehri S, Thawait GK, Williams AA, et al. Imaging characteristics of contralateral asymptomatic patellofemoral joints in patients with unilateral instability. Radiology 2014;273(3):821–30.

34. Best MJ, Tanaka MJ, Demehri S, et al. Accuracy and reliability of the visual assessment of patellar tracking. Am J Sports Med 2020;48(2):370–5.

35. Mousavian A, Shakoor D, Hafezi-Nejad N, et al. Tibiofibular syndesmosis in asymptomatic ankles: initial kinematic analysis using four-dimensional CT. Clin Radiol 2019;74(7):571.e1–8.

36. White J, Couzens G, Jeffery C. The use of 4D-CT in assessing wrist kinematics and pathology: a narrative view. Bone Joint J 2019;101-B(11):1325–30.

37. Zhao K, Breighner R, Holmes D, et al. A technique for quantifying wrist motion using four-dimensional computed tomography: approach and validation. J Biomech Eng 2015;137(7).

38. Leng S, Zhao K, Qu M, et al. Dynamic CT technique for assessment of wrist joint instabilities. Med Phys 2011;38(Suppl 1):S50.

39. Demehri S, Wadhwa V, Thawait GK, et al. Dynamic evaluation of pisotriquetral instability using 4-dimensional computed tomography. J Comput Assist Tomogr 2014;38(4):507–12.

40. Demehri S, Hafezi-Nejad N, Thakur U, et al. Evaluation of pisotriquetral motion pattern using four-dimensional CT: initial clinical experience in asymptomatic wrists. Clin Radiol 2015;70(12):1362–9.

41. Demehri S, Hafezi-Nejad N, Morelli JN, et al. Scapholunate kinematics of asymptomatic wrists in comparison with symptomatic contralateral wrists using four-dimensional CT examinations: initial clinical experience. Skeletal Radiol 2016;45(4):437–46.

42. Shakoor D, Hafezi-Nejad N, Haj-Mirzaian A, et al. Kinematic analysis of the distal radioulnar joint in asymptomatic wrists using 4-dimensional computed tomography-motion pattern and interreader reliability. J Comput Assist Tomogr 2019;43(3):392–8.

43. Totterman SM, Miller R, Wasserman B, et al. Intrinsic and extrinsic carpal ligaments: evaluation by three-dimensional Fourier transform MR imaging. AJR Am J Roentgenol 1993;160(1):117–23.

44. Yoshioka H, Ueno T, Tanaka T, et al. High-resolution MR imaging of triangular fibrocartilage complex (TFCC): comparison of microscopy coils and a conventional small surface coil. Skeletal Radiol 2003; 32(10):575–81.

45. Anderson ML, Skinner JA, Felmlee JP, et al. Diagnostic comparison of 1.5 Tesla and 3.0 Tesla preoperative MRI of the wrist in patients with ulnar-sided wrist pain. J Hand Surg Am 2008;33(7):1153–9.

46. Ochman S, Wieskötter B, Langer M, et al. High-resolution MRI (3T-MRI) in diagnosis of wrist pain: is diagnostic arthroscopy still necessary? Arch Orthop Trauma Surg 2017;137(10):1443–50.

47. Potter HG, Asnis-Ernberg L, Weiland AJ, et al. The utility of high-resolution magnetic resonance imaging in the evaluation of the triangular fibrocartilage complex of the wrist. J Bone Joint Surg Am 1997; 79(11):1675–84.

48. Schmauss D, Pöhlmann S, Lohmeyer JA, et al. Clinical tests and magnetic resonance imaging have limited diagnostic value for triangular fibrocartilaginous complex lesions. Arch Orthop Trauma Surg 2016;136(6):873–80.

49. Iordache SD, Rowan R, Garvin GJ, et al. Prevalence of triangular fibrocartilage complex abnormalities on MRI scans of asymptomatic wrists. J Hand Surg Am 2012;37(1):98–103.

50. De Zwart AD, Beeres FJP, Ring D, et al. MRI as a reference standard for suspected scaphoid fractures. Br J Radiol 2012;85(1016):1098–101.

51. Jeantroux J, Becce F, Guerini H, et al. Athletic injuries of the extensor carpi ulnaris subsheath: MRI findings and utility of gadolinium-enhanced fat-saturated T1-weighted sequences with wrist pronation and supination. Eur Radiol 2011;21(1):160–6.

52. Matloub HS, Dzwierzynski WW, Erickson S, et al. Magnetic resonance imaging scanning in the diagnosis of zone II flexor tendon rupture. J Hand Surg Am 1996;21(3):451–5.

53. Rubin DA, Kneeland JB, Kitay GS, et al. Flexor tendon tears in the hand: use of MR imaging to diagnose degree of injury in a cadaver model. AJR Am J Roentgenol 1996;166(3):615–20.

54. Imaeda T, Nakamura R, Shionoya K, et al. Ulnar impaction syndrome: MR imaging findings. Radiology 1996;201(2):495–500.

55. Maizlin ZV, Brown JA, Clement JJ, et al. MR arthrography of the wrist: controversies and concepts. Hand (N Y) 2009;4(1):66–73.

56. Scheck RJ, Kubitzek C, Hierner R, et al. The scapholunate interosseous ligament in MR arthrography of the wrist: correlation with non-enhanced MRI and wrist arthroscopy. Skeletal Radiol 1997;26(5):263–71.

57. Schweitzer ME, Natale P, Winalski CS, et al. Indirect wrist MR arthrography: the effects of passive motion versus active exercise. Skeletal Radiol 2000;29(1):10–4.

58. Haims AH, Schweitzer ME, Morrison WB, et al. Internal derangement of the wrist: indirect MR

arthrography versus unenhanced MR imaging. Radiology 2003;227(3):701–7.

59. Pfirrmann CWA, Zanetti M. Variants, pitfalls and asymptomatic findings in wrist and hand imaging. Eur J Radiol 2005;56(3):286–95.

60. Reid M, Wood T, Montgomery A-M, et al. MRI does not effectively diagnose ulnar-sided wrist pain in elite tennis players. J Sci Med Sport 2020;23(6): 564–8.

61. Jedlinski A, Kauer JM, Jonsson K. X-ray evaluation of the true neutral position of the wrist: the groove for extensor carpi ulnaris as a landmark. J Hand Surg Am 1995;20(3):511–2.

62. Yang Z, Mann FA, Gilula LA, et al. Scaphopisocapitate alignment: criterion to establish a neutral lateral view of the wrist. Radiology 1997;205(3):865–9.

63. Goldfarb CA, Yin Y, Gilula LA, et al. Wrist fractures: what the clinician wants to know. Radiology 2001; 219(1):11–28.

64. May MM, Lawton JN, Blazar PE. Ulnar styloid fractures associated with distal radius fractures: incidence and implications for distal radioulnar joint instability. J Hand Surg Am 2002;27(6):965–71.

65. Nakamura T, Iwamoto T, Matsumura N, et al. Radiographic and arthroscopic assessment of DRUJ instability due to foveal avulsion of the radioulnar ligament in distal radius fractures. J Wrist Surg 2014; 3(1):12–7.

Extensor Carpi Ulnaris Subluxation

Jacqueline N. Byrd, MD, MPH[a,b], Sarah E. Sasor, MD[c], Kevin C. Chung, MD, MS[a,*]

KEYWORDS

- Hand surgery • Wrist pain • Patient outcomes • Sports injuries

KEY POINTS

- The subsheath is vulnerable to tears in acute wrist movements, especially those combining supination, flexion, and ulnar deviation.
- Surgical repair with a flap of extensor retinaculum to re-create the tendon's stabilizing subsheath is recommended.

BACKGROUND

Extensor carpi ulnaris (ECU) subluxation is an increasingly recognized cause of ulnar-sided wrist pain. The ECU tendon runs in the ulnar groove and is stabilized within a fibroosseus tunnel. A subsheath acts as labrum on the ulnar border of the ulnar groove and prevents subluxation. Subsheath tears can occur with resisted forearm supination, wrist flexion, and ulnar deviation. Injuries are most common in athletes who play racquet or stick sports.[1] ECU subluxation also occurs in rheumatoid patients owing to synovitis and attenuation of the subsheath.[2] This article reviews pertinent anatomy, diagnosis, and management of ECU subluxation.

ANATOMY

The ECU originates at the lateral epicondyle of the humerus and inserts on the base of the fifth metacarpal. At the wrist level, it runs within the sixth dorsal compartment and is stabilized by a distinct subsheath (**Fig. 1**). The subsheath is deep to the extensor retinaculum and maintains the tendon within the ulnar groove: it acts as a labrum along the ulnar side of the groove and prevents tendon subluxation. The subsheath lacks elastic fibers and is resistant to rupture. It is reinforced by the *linea jugata*, a sling of collagen fibers that inserts onto the interosseus membrane.

PATHOPHYSIOLOGY

ECU tendinopathies are classified as constrained or unconstrained.[3] In constrained tendinopathy, the subsheath is too tight and restricts tendon gliding; this causes pain and dysfunction.[4] Unconstrained tendinopathy occurs if the subsheath is torn or attenuated, and the tendon subluxates around the ulnar head.[3] Both tendinopathies produce ulnar-sided wrist pain. A careful history and physical examination can help differentiate between the two.

The ECU is under maximal stress when the wrist is supinated, flexed, and ulnarly deviated. If the subsheath tears, the ECU subluxates volarly and ulnarly over the ulnar head. Sudden, forceful contraction of the ECU or repetitive, minor trauma causes attenuation of both the tendon and the subsheath.[2,5] It may be necessary to treat both the subsheath and the tendon during surgery.[4]

[a] Section of Plastic Surgery, Department of Surgery, University of Michigan Medical School, North Campus Research Complex, 2800 Plymouth Road, Building 16, Room 122W, Ann Arbor, MI 48109, USA; [b] Department of Surgery, University of Texas Southwestern Medical School, Dallas, TX, USA; [c] Department of Plastic Surgery, Medical College of Wisconsin, Tosa Center, South Entry, Suite T2500, 1155 N Mayfair Road, Wauwatosa, WI 53226, USA
* Corresponding author. Section of Plastic Surgery, University of Michigan Comprehensive Hand Center, The University of Michigan Health System, 1500 East Medical Center Drive, 2130 Taubman Center, SPC 5340, Ann Arbor, MI 48109-5340.
E-mail address: kecchung@med.umich.edu

Hand Clin 37 (2021) 487–491
https://doi.org/10.1016/j.hcl.2021.06.005
0749-0712/21/© 2021 Elsevier Inc. All rights reserved.

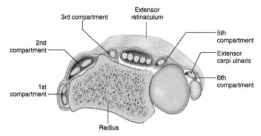

Fig. 1. Sixth dorsal compartment. (*From* Sears ED, Fujihara N, Chung KC. Stabilization of Extensor Carpi Ulnaris TendonSubluxation with Extensor Retinaculum. In: Chung KC, ed. *Operative Techniques: Hand and Wrist Surgery.* Elsevier; 2018:636 to 641; with permission.)

Tears to the subsheath are classified into 3 types (**Fig. 2**). Type A is the most common and occurs at the ulnar side of the subsheath. The tendon is able to return to the ulna groove under the torn edge of subsheath. Type B tears occur at the radial side of the sheath and are less likely to heal, as the tendon lies outside of the torn sheath. The third class, type C, occurs when the fibrous subsheath is detached from the ulna's periosteum. With this widened subsheath, the tendon can move out of the ulnar groove and remain in a false sheath.[1] Understanding the classification of subsheath tears is important when evaluating a new patient, as some tears are unlikely to heal with conservative management.[5]

PHYSICAL EXAMINATION

ECU subluxation can be a challenging diagnosis. Patients may present to an athletic trainer or primary care provider before referral to a hand surgeon. It is important that providers who treat at-risk athletes are aware of its presenting signs and symptoms. Patients with an acute injury present with swelling, tenderness, and pain over the dorsal ulnar wrist. In the chronic setting, tendon snapping and wrist instability may be present.

The ECU synergy and subluxation tests are helpful diagnostic maneuvers.[6,7] To perform the ECU synergy test, the patient supinates the wrist, and the examiner applies resistance at the radial side of the hand. The patient's elbow should be resting on the table, the wrist neutral, and the fingers extended (**Fig. 3**). This position provokes isometric contraction of the ECU and flexor carpi ulnaris muscles. The test is positive for a constrained ECU tendinopathy if the patient has pain. The examiner may palpate bowstringing of the tendon if there is subluxation. The synergy test has been shown to predict ECU tendon abnormalities when compared with sonographic evaluation. Sato and colleagues[8] found the ECU synergy test had a sensitivity of 74% and specificity of 86%.

To perform the ECU subluxation test, the patient supinates while the examiner applies resistance to the ulnar aspect of the hand. The patient is then asked to ulnarly deviate the wrist. This test should be performed by the examiner on both wrists for comparison of asymptomatic subluxation.[6] Another test to evaluate both wrists simultaneously is the "heart-like test." In this test, the backs of the hands are placed together against the chest with the thumbs pointed up. This provoking maneuver can produce the snapping sound and sensation.[3]

IMAGING

Wrist radiographs are mandatory to rule out bony pathologic condition. Because of its superficial location, the ECU tendon can be assessed with ultrasonography. This must be used in conjunction with the patient's history, as this dynamic imaging can also identify ECU subsheath instability in asymptomatic patients. MRI can be used to characterize the anatomy of the tendon and the ulnar groove, but it is not routine in preoperative planning.[9]

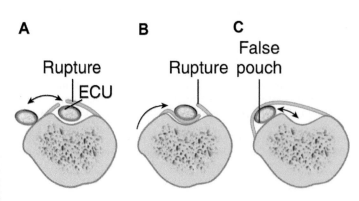

Fig. 2. Classification of subsheath tears as type A, B, or C. (*From* Sears ED, Fujihara N, Chung KC. Stabilization. of Extensor Carpi Ulnaris Tendon Subluxation with Extensor Retinaculum. In: Chung KC, ed. *Operative Techniques: Hand and Wrist Surgery.* Elsevier; 2018:636 to 641; with permission.)

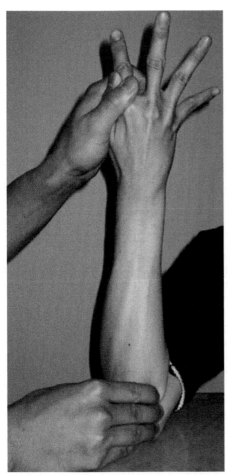

Fig. 3. The ECU synergy test. (*From* Sears ED, Fujihara N, Chung KC. Stabilization of Extensor Carpi Ulnaris Tendon Subluxation with Extensor Retinaculum. In: Chung KC, ed. *Operative Techniques: Hand and Wrist Surgery.* Elsevier; 2018:636 to 641; with permission.)

TREATMENT

Initial management is immobilization in a long-arm cast for 6 weeks. Surgery is indicated for patients who continue to have pain or instability after a trial of immobilization.

Surgical Options

In the acute setting, primary subsheath repair may be possible. This assessment is made intraoperatively based on the injury and involved tissue. The torn subsheath can be debrided and repaired in some acute type A and B tears. In the acute type C tear, a similar primary repair would be reattaching the avulsed periosteum to close the sheath over the tendon.[3] For chronic injuries, reconstruction of the subsheath is often necessary. There are multiple techniques using flaps of extensor

retinaculum with or without bone anchors. The authors' preferred technique is to use an ulnarly based flap to create a sling for the ECU tendon. This reconstruction was first reported by Spinner and Kaplan.[2] The only contraindication is a history of prior wrist surgeries with scarring of the extensor retinaculum.[10]

Surgical Technique

The surgery is performed under general anesthesia or an axillary nerve block with a tourniquet. A 5-cm incision over the dorsal ulnar wrist is made for exposure (**Fig. 4**). The dorsal sensory branch of the ulnar nerve runs in the subcutaneous tissue in this area and must be avoided. The extensor retinaculum over the sixth compartment is incised to expose the ECU tendon. The torn edges of the subsheath and any frayed tendon are debrided. If the subsheath edges come together without tension, a primary repair can be performed at this stage. If proceeding with subsheath reconstruction, a 3-cm wide flap is planned (**Fig. 5**). The flap is based at the ulnar border of the fifth extensor compartment. The radial limit is the radial aspect of the third compartment. The flap is carefully elevated from radial to ulnar.

The ECU tendon is then carefully mobilized from the damaged subsheath. The flap of extensor retinaculum is passed under the ECU tendon (**Fig. 6**). The flap is wrapped around the tendon and sutured to itself with 2-0 Ethibond sutures (**Fig. 7**). These sutures control the size of the new ECU tendon sheath. It is important to assess the relationship of the ECU tendon and the new subsheath. If this is too tight, the patient can develop ECU tendonitis postoperatively. If it is too lax, the wrist will continue to be symptomatic. Additional sutures can be placed to anchor the flap to the adjacent extensor retinaculum.[11]

If there is concern for other wrist pathologic conditions, one can perform wrist arthroscopy during the same procedure. Wrist arthroscopy is both diagnostic and potentially therapeutic, minimizing the risk of reoperation for unaddressed second pathologic condition. Half (8 out of 15) of the flap repairs done in the published series from Massachusetts General Hospital required an additional surgery. The most common was tenosynovectomy (4 out of 8 combination cases), followed by triangular fibrocartilage complex repair (2 of 8 combination cases).[4] A similar observation was made in a series from Austria. Of 12 patients undergoing ECU extensor retinaculum flap reconstruction, 6 had isolated ECU pathologic condition. Other surgeries performed at the time of the flap ranged from arthroscopy to ulnar shortening.[12]

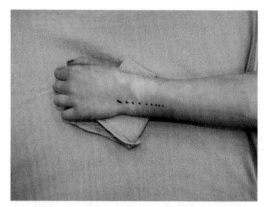

Fig. 4. Planned incision for ECU reconstruction.

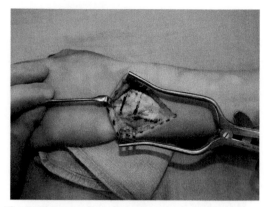

Fig. 5. Planning flap of extensor retinaculum.

Postoperatively, patients are placed in a long-arm splint with the wrist in neutral for 4 to 6 weeks. Patients should avoid strenuous physical activities for 3 months.[11] Although single-center studies vary in technique and have small samples, recurrence of symptomatic subluxation and ECU tendon rupture is rare.[1,4,10,12] Some patients may experience postoperative tendinitis[4]; this could be due to residual tendinopathy, but it underscores the need for careful sizing of the reconstructed ECU sheath.

DISCUSSION

Subsheath reconstruction with the extensor retinaculum flap has high rates of patient satisfaction.[4,10,12] A single-center series published in 2020 found no recurrent subluxation.[4] If MRI is used to confirm the diagnosis, it can be used to compare postoperative results. A group in Austria published a series of 12 patients with preoperative and postoperative MRI findings. The investigators reported 4 patients with persistent ECU dislocation on repeat MRI. However, these patients all reported excellent satisfaction with the surgery.[12] Although this is a small study, it suggests the cause for ulnar wrist pain may not be the action of tendon dislocation. This finding is supported by the radiologic findings of subluxation in asymptomatic wrists.[13] In addition, a cadaveric study identified ECU subluxation with intact subsheath.[14] The resolution of pain after reconstruction of the sheath suggests the relationship between subluxation and pain is more complex.

Research continues to support and refine surgical approaches. The ulnar groove can be deepened with a bur if it is too shallow, but there is no evidence to support routine deepening. A cadaveric model evaluating routine deepening of the ulnar groove did not find increased stability of the repair.[15] Understanding the underlying biomechanics of the ECU tendon-subsheath complex is vital to improving surgical outcomes. Current studies highlight opportunities to further investigate the cause of ulnar-sided wrist pain associated with tendon subluxation.

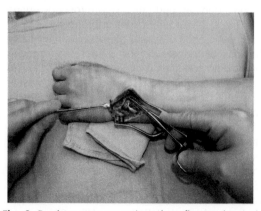

Fig. 6. Passing extensor retinaculum flap under and over the ECU tendon.

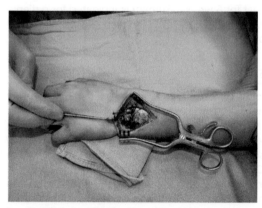

Fig. 7. The completed reconstruction of the ECU sheath with a flap of extensor retinaculum.

SUMMARY

The unique function of the ECU subsheath serves to stabilize the wrist during movements. Damage to the subsheath can result from sports injuries or traumatic movement and produces ulnar-sided wrist pain. Conservative management allows for anatomic healing in only some causes of subluxation. Surgical repair facilitates return to sports and function.

CLINICS CARE POINTS

- Extensor carpi ulnaris subluxation can be a challenging diagnosis as a cause of wrist pain.
- Surgery is indicated for patients who do not respond to conservative measures.
- If possible, a tension-free repair of the torn subsheath should be performed.
- A flap of extensor retinaculum can be used to re-create the extensor carpi ulnaris subsheath with good long-term outcome.

DISCLOSURE

Funding: J.N. Byrd is supported by a Surgical Scientist Training Grant in Health Services and Translational Research (5 T32 GM 8616-20) from the National Institutes of Health Ruth L. Kirschstein National Research Service Award.

Financial Disclosure: None of the authors has a financial interest in any of the drugs, products, or devices mentioned in this discussion or the manuscript being discussed.

REFERENCES

1. Inoue G, Tamura Y. Surgical treatment for recurrent dislocation of the extensor carpi ulnaris tendon. J Hand Surg Br 2001;26(6):556–9.
2. Spinner M, Kaplan EB. Extensor carpi ulnaris. Its relationship to the stability of the distal radio-ulnar joint. Clin Orthop Relat Res 1970;68:124–9.
3. Garcia-Elias M. Tendinopathies of the extensor carpi ulnaris. Handchir Mikrochir Plast Chir 2015;47(5):281–9.
4. Verhiel S, Ozkan S, Chen NC, et al. Long-term outcomes after extensor carpi ulnaris subsheath reconstruction with extensor retinaculum. Tech Hand Up Extrem Surg 2020;24(1):2–6.
5. Inoue G, Tamura Y. Recurrent dislocation of the extensor carpi ulnaris tendon. Br J Sports Med 1998;32(2):172–4.
6. Garcia-Elias M. Clinical examination of the ulnar-sided painful wrist. In: del Piñal F, editor. Arthroscopic management of ulnar pain. Berlin, Heidelberg: Springer Berlin Heidelberg; 2012. p. 25–44.
7. Ruland RT, Hogan CJ. The ECU synergy test: an aid to diagnose ECU tendonitis. J Hand Surg Am 2008;33(10):1777–82.
8. Sato J, Ishii Y, Noguchi H. Diagnostic performance of the extensor carpi ulnaris (ECU) synergy test to detect sonographic ECU abnormalities in chronic dorsal ulnar-sided wrist pain. J Ultrasound Med 2016;35(1):7–14.
9. Dineen HA, Greenberg JA. Ulnar-sided wrist pain in the athlete. Clin Sports Med 2020;39(2):373–400.
10. MacLennan AJ, Nemechek NM, Waitayawinyu T, et al. Diagnosis and anatomic reconstruction of extensor carpi ulnaris subluxation. J Hand Surg Am 2008;33(1):59–64.
11. Sears EDF N, Chung KC. Stabilization of extensor carpi ulnaris tendon subluxation with extensor retinaculum. In: Chung KC, editor. Operative techniques: hand and wrist surgery. Philadelphia: Elsevier; 2018. p. 636–41.
12. Peter K, Luzian H, Markus G, et al. Mid-term outcome (11-90 months) of the extensor retinaculum flap procedure for extensor carpi ulnaris tendon instability. Arch Orthop Trauma Surg 2019;139(9):1323–8.
13. Sole JS, Wisniewski SJ, Newcomer KL, et al. Sonographic evaluation of the extensor carpi ulnaris in asymptomatic tennis players. PM R 2015;7(3):255–63.
14. Ghatan AC, Puri SG, Morse KW, et al. Relative contribution of the subsheath to extensor carpi ulnaris tendon stability: implications for surgical reconstruction and rehabilitation. J Hand Surg Am 2016;41(2):225–32.
15. Puri SK, Morse KW, Hearns KA, et al. A biomechanical comparison of extensor carpi ulnaris subsheath reconstruction techniques. J Hand Surg 2017;42(10):837.e831–7.

Triangular Fibrocartilage Complex Repair/Reconstruction

Lauren M. Shapiro, MD, MS[a], Jeffrey Yao, MD[b],*

KEYWORDS

- Triangular fibrocartilage complex reconstruction • Triangular fibrocartilage complex repair
- Triangular fibrocartilage complex tear • Ulnar-sided wrist pain

KEY POINTS

- A thorough understanding of the complex anatomy, vascularization, and nuances of the physical examination of the TFCC are required to understand and guide treatment
- Treatment of TFCC injuries includes arthroscopic, arthroscopic-assisted, and open techniques that are typically determined by the injury pattern and surgeon experience
- Outcomes of repair and reconstruction vary by technique; however, when utilized for the appropriate indications, demonstrate reliable improvement in pain, stability, range of motion, and disability

INTRODUCTION/HISTORY/DEFINITIONS/BACKGROUND

The triangular fibrocartilage complex (TFCC) plays an important role at the distal radioulnar joint (DRUJ) by providing stability and serving as a shock absorber and load transmitter.[1–4] Given the functional role of the ulnar wrist and its use in many activities of daily living and athletics, injuries of the TFCC are common.[5–7] Injuries may occur in isolation or in combination with other wrist or intracarpal pathologies (eg, distal radius fractures). Given the complexity of the DRUJ, the diagnosis and treatment of a TFCC injury may present as a diagnostic challenge. In this article, we aim to illustrate the anatomy, diagnosis, classification systems, approaches to, treatment management, and outcomes of TFCC injuries requiring repair or reconstruction.

NATURE OF THE PROBLEM/DIAGNOSIS

TFCC tears classically occur with an extension and pronation force to an axially loaded wrist. These injuries are commonly seen with a fall from a height with a twisting moment placed on the wrist. These injuries are the most common cause of ulnar-sided wrist pain, and chronic injuries may lead to persistent pain and possible DRUJ instability and arthritis. Although the full physical examination of the ulnar side of the wrist has been discussed in a prior article in this issue, we briefly highlight the salient examination maneuvers specific to TFCC injury. The authors typically perform the following maneuvers: TFCC grind test, fovea sign, the "frying pan" sign, pain with hypersupination/hyperpronation, and we evaluate for DRUJ stability (**Table 1**).

ANATOMY

The anatomy of the TFCC is intricate, yet its understanding is critical to guide diagnosis and treatment. It is composed of the triangular fibrocartilage articular disc (TFC), the ulnar collateral ligament (UCL), the extensor carpi ulnaris (ECU) subsheath, and the superficial and deep

[a] Department of Orthopaedic Surgery, Duke University, 4709 Creekstone Drive, Durham, NC 27703, USA;
[b] Department of Orthopaedic Surgery, Stanford University, 450 Broadway Street, MC: 6120, Redwood City, CA 94603, USA
* Corresponding author.
E-mail address: jyao@stanford.edu

Hand Clin 37 (2021) 493–505
https://doi.org/10.1016/j.hcl.2021.06.006

Table 1
Specific physical examination maneuvers for evaluating the TFCC

Exam/Maneuver	Technique	Significance
TFCC grind test[a]	The examiner ulnarly deviates the wrist and moves the wrist through a flexion/extension arc in ulnar deviation.	The examination maneuver is positive if this motion recreates the patient's pain.
Fovea sign[a]	The examiner places his or her thumb into the interval between the ulnar styloid and FCU tendon between the volar ulnar head and the pisiform	The examination maneuver is positive if this pressure recreates the patient's pain.
The "frying pan" sign	The examiner places a heavy object (such as a JAMAR grip meter or something similar) into the wrist to simulate the weight of a frying pan with a long lever arm placing the wrist into in hypersupination that simulates the pain. Patients also frequently report they are unable to carry a heavy frying pan because of their symptoms.	The examination maneuver is positive if this recreates the patient's pain.
Ballottement test[a]	The examiner stabilizes the radius with 2 fingers of one hand and moves the ulna both volar and dorsal with 2 fingers from the other hand. The amount of displacement is evaluated relative to the contralateral side in pronation, neutral, and supination.	This examination maneuver is positive if the displacement in pronation, neutral, or supination is greater than that of the contralateral side.
Hypersupination and pronation	The maneuver is performed with the patient's elbows at the side of their body. The patient is asked to point their thumb up. The patient is asked to supinate and pronate their forearm. This is measured relative to the contralateral side.	This examination maneuver is positive if there is pain with hypersupination or hyperpronation.

Abbreviations: FCU, flexor carpi ulnaris; TFCC, triangular fibrocartilage complex.
[a] These maneuvers/tests are performed with the patient's elbow in 90° with the elbow resting on the examination table.

volar and dorsal radioulnar ligaments[8] (**Fig. 1**). The superficial and deep layers are discrete and insert/become confluent with the ECU subsheath and the fovea/base of the ulnar styloid, respectively.

The vascular supply of the TFCC also helps to guide treatment. Cadaveric studies have demonstrated that the TFCC is supplied by the ulnar artery and the palmar and dorsal branches of the anterior interosseous artery that provide vessels from the peripheral capsule and synovial tissue that penetrate the TFCC in a radial fashion and supply the peripheral 10% to 40% of the TFCC.[9] Thiru and colleagues[10] demonstrated vascularity of the peripheral 15% to 20% of the TFCC. Although the exact extent of vascularity likely demonstrates some variation, the lack of a vascular supply centrally has negative implications for healing potential and thus success of attempted repair (**Fig. 2**).

Current classification schemes help provide a framework for understanding the injury and for communicating the nature of the injury to other providers. Palmer[11] classified TFCC injuries into broad categories of traumatic (Class 1) or degenerative (Class 2), the former of which are further categorized based on injury location. Class 1A involves tears that are central in location and include an isolated central disk perforation, Class 1B are peripheral, ulnar-sided tears (with or without an ulnar styloid fracture), Class 1C are distal TFCC injuries that typically involve disruption of the TFCC from the distal ulnocarpal ligaments, Class 1D tears are radial sided tears that may or may not include a fracture of the sigmoid notch[11] (**Fig. 3**). Degenerative tears (Class 2) are typically a result of chronic and/or excessive loading through the ulnolunate joint, commonly seen in

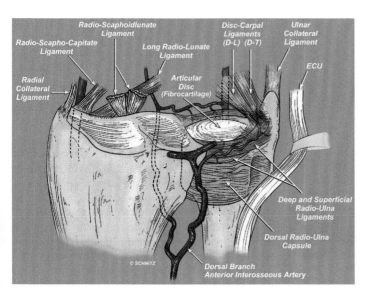

Fig. 1. Anatomic illustration of the triangular fibrocartilage complex and its components. (*From* Kleinman WB. Stability of the Distal Radioulna Joint: Biomechanics, Pathophysiology, Physical Diagnosis, and Restoration of Function What We Have Learned in 25 Years. J Hand Surg Am. 2007;32(7):1086-106; with permission.)

patients with ulnar positive variance and ulnar impaction syndrome. These degenerative injuries are typically less amenable to repair or reconstruction, are treated with simple debridement and/or ulnar leveling procedures, and are therefore outside of the scope of this article.

Atzei and colleagues[12] created a classification schema further describing peripheral TFCC injuries with a treatment-oriented approach. The investigators first divide the TFCC into 3 principal structures: (1) the proximal triangular ligament (the ligamentum subcruentum), (2) the distal hammock structure (the superficial radioulnar ligament), and (3) the UCL and subsequently describe 5 injury classes with corresponding treatment recommendations[12,13] (**Fig. 4**).

Class 0 injuries include an isolated ulnar styloid fracture without a TFCC injury. These patients demonstrate no instability of the DRUJ. During arthroscopy, the TFCC appears normal and is taught (unable to be hooked with a probe, ie, negative hook test). Symptomatic immobilization is the mainstay of treatment. Fragment excision may be performed for refractory ulnar wrist pain. Class 1

Dorsal branch of anterior interosseous artery

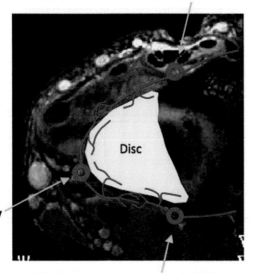

Ulnar artery

Palmar branch of anterior interosseous artery

Fig. 2. Illustration of the vascular supply of the triangular fibrocartilage complex. (*From* Vezeridis, P.S., Yoshioka, H., Han, R. et al. Ulnar-sided wrist pain. Part I: anatomy and physical examination. Skeletal Radiol 39, 733–745 (2010). https://doi.org/10.1007/s00256-009-0775-x.)

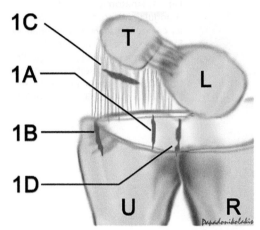

Fig. 3. Illustration of the traumatic or Class 1 Palmer classification. (*From* Chloros GD, Wiesler ER, Poehling GG. Current Concepts in Wrist Arthroscopy. Arthroscopy.2008;24(3):343-54; with permission.)

injuries involve a distal TFCC tear with slight DRUJ laxity. During arthroscopy, the distal TFCC may have a peripheral tear; however, the hook test is negative. Treatment for Class 1 injuries includes suturing the TFCC back to the ulnar capsule ("capsular repair"). Class 2 injuries comprise complete TFCC injuries, including the peripheral and deep portions. These patients may demonstrate

mild to severe laxity with a soft endpoint. The distal TFCC from the arthroscope appears normal; however, the hook test is positive. Treatment involves foveal reinsertion of the TFCC in these cases. Class 3 injuries include those with a proximal TFCC tear, mild to severe laxity of the DRUJ with a soft endpoint, and a normal-appearing TFCC on radiocarpal arthroscopy with a positive hook test. Similar to Class 2 injuries, Class 3 injuries may be better diagnosed with DRUJ arthroscopy and are treated with foveal reinsertion unless they are accompanied by a basilar ulnar styloid fracture (which represents an avulsion injury of the TFCC insertion). In these cases (subclassified as 3A), ulnar styloid fixation (with cannulated screws, tension band wiring, k-wires) is recommended. Class 4 injuries include nonrepairable TFCC tears. Two subclassifications exist, Class 4A is consistent with a massive tear with degenerated edges, whereas Class 4B is associated with a TFCC with frayed edges or a previously failed TFCC suture repair. Class 4A and 4B are differentiated primarily based on why they are irreparable (4A has a sizable defect, 4B has poor healing capacity). These patients present with mild to severe TFCC laxity with a soft endpoint and all have a positive hook test. The mainstay of treatment for 4A and 4B injuries is a tendon graft reconstruction. Class 5 are those patients demonstrating DRUJ

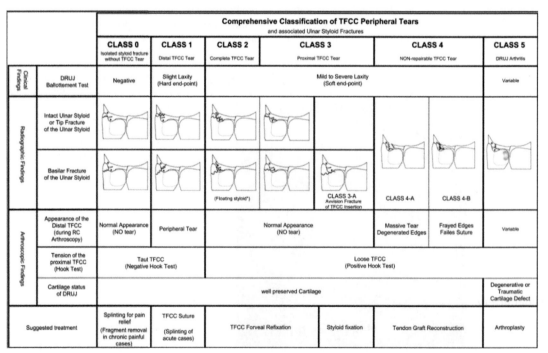

Fig. 4. Atzei and colleagues[12] classification schema describing TFCC classification with corresponding clinical, imaging, arthroscopic findings, and treatment recommendations. (*From* Atzei A, Luchetti R. Foveal TFCC tear classification and treatment. Hand Clin. 2011;27(3):263-272; with permission.)

arthritis. The amount of instability and appearance of the TFCC with the arthroscope are variable. These patients are typically indicated for an arthroplasty procedure.

PREOPERATIVE/PREPROCEDURE PLANNING

Appropriate understanding of the injury, any concomitant injuries, and any factors underlying the pathophysiology are critical to ensure a successful procedure. It is important to evaluate and recognize the variance of the ulna, the presence of ulnar abutment, DRUJ instability, articular incongruity or arthritis, and the presence of any skeletal deformities. Although outside the scope of this article, the presence of these may influence treatment (ie, the addition of an ulnar shortening osteotomy).

The authors typically start with immobilization as first-line treatment for any TFCC tear that does not demonstrate instability. Immobilization is supplemented with activity modification, anti-inflammatory medications, and/or corticosteroid injections as needed. Park and colleagues[14] retrospectively evaluated a cohort of patients with a TFCC injury and demonstrated symptomatic relief in 57% of patients after 4 weeks of immobilization. The optimal interval of immobilization and a cost-effective analysis of an appropriate time of immobilization are not known. Patients with stable TFCC injuries who have failed immobilization after 4 weeks may be surgical candidates.

Surgical options for TFCC tears typically fall within the categories of debridement, repair, and reconstruction. Debridement is typically used for central and radial tears given the lack of vascularity and thus less robust healing potential. Exceptions do exist, however, when there is a residual cuff of TFCC that may be repairable or more importantly if there is any concomitant DRUJ instability. In the case of DRUJ instability, repair should be considered and/or attempted when possible.

Due to the rich vascularity of the periphery of the TFCC complex, injuries here are the most amenable to healing and are thus most amenable to repair. For the purposes of this discussion, we focus on the tears that are most amenable to repair or reconstruction: the peripheral tears (Palmer 1B). Peripheral tears and/or tears resulting in DRUJ instability (eg, disruption of the foveal attachment) should be treated with repair. Reconstruction is reserved for irreparable TFCC tears due to poor tissue quality or large irreparable tears with evidence of DRUJ instability. Given the scope of this article, we discuss arthroscopic and open techniques for repair and reconstruction of peripheral (Palmer 1B) TFCC tears.

PREPARATION AND PATIENT POSITIONING

The decision between treatment with arthroscopic versus arthroscopic-assisted versus open TFCC treatment techniques is mainly guided by surgeon training, experience, and comfort level with these techniques. Investigations have essentially shown equivalent outcomes between these techniques. However, arthroscopic methods minimize soft tissue trauma, allow for examination of the entire joint for concomitant pathology, and may provide a more rapid recovery.[15–20] When an arthroscopic technique or an arthroscopic-assisted technique is used, preparation and positioning for a standard wrist arthroscopic procedure are used. A hand table and a sterile traction device with approximately 12 to 15 lb of traction are used. A 2.7-mm to 3.5-mm 30° arthroscope is typically used. For an open repair or reconstruction, a hand table is also used. A tourniquet is used for both arthroscopic and open procedures.

PROCEDURAL APPROACH FOR CAPSULAR REPAIR

This approach describes an arthroscopic capsular repair technique for a Palmer type 1B superficial tear (Atzei Class 1 peripheral tears).

- Inflate tourniquet
- Identify and create the 3-4 portal (1 cm distal to Listers tubercle)
- Identify and create the 6R portal (just radial to ECU)
- Identify and debride the peripheral tear to stimulate an angiogenic healing response
- Perform a traditional outside-in arthroscopic-assisted TFCC repair[17,21]:
  - A 1-cm incision is made at the 6R portal, blunt dissection is used to avoid nerve injury, and an up to 50% incision in the retinaculum over the ECU is performed
  - With the ECU retracted, a cannulated needle is inserted through the floor of the sixth extensor compartment, starting proximal to the disc and penetrating the disc from proximal to distal under arthroscopic visualization
  - A wire loop of the retriever is placed over the needle, a 2-0 or 3-0 PDS suture is inserted, and the needle and retriever are extracted leaving the suture in place
  - These steps are repeated 2 to 4 times, consistent with the number of sutures needed
  - The forearm is placed in slight supination to reduce tension on the defect, and the sutures are pulled taught to bring the articular

disc to the dorsal capsule, and tied over the floor of the sixth extensor compartment underneath the ECU

- **Fig. 5** illustrates the step-by-step technique and final construct
- Alternatively, our preference for an all-arthroscopic capsular repair[15]:
  - With the arthroscope in the 6R portal, a curved TFCC FasT-Fix (Smith and Nephew Endoscopy, Andover, MA) is inserted into the 3 to 4 portal with the assistance of the splint cannula
  - The first limb of the FasT-Fix (the poly-L-lactate [PLLA] block) is advanced through the articular disc, traversing the tear and then passed through the ulnar capsule
  - After penetration of the capsule (noted by a decrease in resistance), the trigger is deployed on the needle introducer to release the first PLLA block onto the outside of the ulnar capsule. The needle introducer is drawn back into the radio-carpal joint and advanced to the ulnar side of the tear
  - The second PLLA block is placed in the same manner just ulnar to the tear, forming a vertical mattress configuration

- The needle introducer is removed and the 2-0 pre-tied suture is tightened and cut with a knot pusher and cutter, respectively
- A second TFCC FasT-Fix may be used if needed for improved reduction/repair
- **Fig. 6** illustrates the step-by-step technique and final construct

PROCEDURAL APPROACH FOR FOVEAL REPAIR

This approach describes the authors' preferred arthroscopic foveal repair technique for a Palmer type 1B deep or complete tear (Atzei Class 2 or 3 peripheral tears). Of note, the arthroscopic and arthroscopic-assisted techniques have many iterations, particularly with regard to anchoring the TFCC to the fovea.[22–24]

- Inflate the tourniquet.
- Identify and create the 3 to 4 portal (1 cm distal to the Lister tubercle).
- Identify and create the 6R portal (just radial to the ECU).
- Identify and debride the foveal tear.
- Make a 1-cm incision 1.5 cm proximal to the ulnar styloid along the subcutaneous border of the ulna.

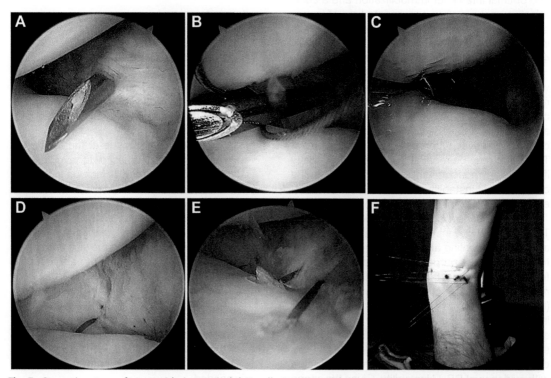

Fig. 5. Operative steps of an outside-in repair. (*A*) Needle insertion, (*B*) wire suture insertion, (*C*) PDS suture insertion, (*D*) first suture placed, (*E*) final construct with 2 sutures placed, (*F*) knots are tied over the floor of the sixth extensor compartment. (*From* Papapetropoulos PA, Ruch DS. Repair of Arthroscopic Triangular Fibrocartilage Complex Tears in Athletes. Hand Clin. 2009;25(3):389-94; with permission.)

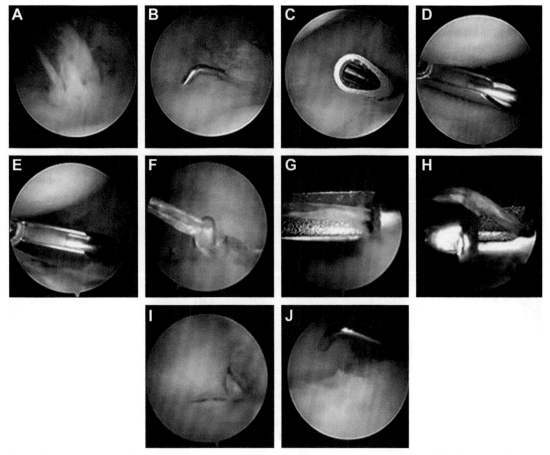

Fig. 6. Operative steps of an all inside repair. (A) Tear identification and classification, (B) demonstration of a negative trampoline effect, (C) tear debridement, (D) FasT-fix suture inserted through the 3 to 4 portal, (E) second FasT-fix suture inserted, (F) needle introducer is removed leaving the pretied suture, (G) suture tightened with a knot pusher, (H) suture cut with a knot cutter, (I) final construct demonstrating repair, (J) demonstration of a negative trampoline effect. (*From* Yao J. All-arthroscopic repair of peripheral triangular fibrocartilage complex tears using FasT-Fix. Hand Clin. 2011;27(3):237-42; with permission.)

- Insert a 2.0 mm guidewire from outside in from the ulnar neck exiting through the fovea, underneath the articular disc. This step is done under arthroscopic (viewing from the 3–4 portal) and fluoroscopic visualization and guidance.
- Drill over this wire with a cannulated 3.0-mm drill.
- Place a 4-0 Fiberstick (Arthrex, Naples, FL) suture on a suture passer (Arthrex) through the articular disc of the TFCC under arthroscopic visualization.
- Using a suture loop, the end of the repair suture is pulled through the articular disc of the TFCC a second time and subsequently passed back down the osseous tunnel.
- Instruments inserted into the 6R or 6U portal may assist in this process.
- The sutures are pulled taught, reduction of the tear is arthroscopically evaluated, and the sutures are tied onto the ulnar periosteum or inserted into a knotless suture anchor (Arthrex PushLok, Naples, FL) and embedded into a drillhole created in the proximal ulna.
- This technique may be repeated to place multiple sutures.
- **Fig. 7** illustrates the technique and final construct described.

The following approach describes an open foveal repair technique for a Palmer type 1B deep or complete tear (Atzei Class 2 or 3 peripheral tears).[23]

- Inflate the tourniquet.
- Make a dorsally based, longitudinal incision between the fifth and sixth extensor compartments, centered over the ulnar head.
- Open the fifth extensor compartment and retract the extensor digiti minimi tendon ulnarly, exposing the dorsal DRUJ capsule.

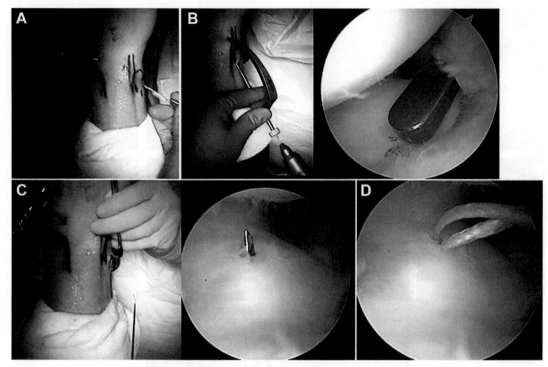

Fig. 7. Arthroscopic repair of a foveal tear. (*A*) With the arthroscope in the 3 to 4 portal, a 1.5-cm longitudinal incision is made proximal to the ulnar styloid. (*B*) A guidewire is placed from outside in from the ulnar neck exiting the fovea (this step is done under arthroscopic and fluoroscopic visualization and guidance and may be assisted with a C-clamp guide. (*C*) Fiberstick suture (Arthrex, Naples, FL) is placed via a suture passer under arthroscopic visualization. (*D*) Sutures are shuttled through before being tied down or inserted into a knotless suture anchor on the ulna.

- The foveal tear may be visualized by making a 3-cm L-shaped incision along the neck of the ulna and proximal to the dorsal distal radioulnar ligament.
- Scar tissue about the fovea is debrided and 2 pilot holes are made near the center of the fovea with a 1.2-mm k-wire.
- Two sutures (nylon or polyester) are passed through the holes from the fovea to the lateral ulnar cortex and tied over the bone bridge.
  - Alternatively, suture anchor(s) may be placed into the fovea to be used for the repair.
- The radioulnar ligament is sutured back with a locking mattress technique.
- The extensor digiti minimi tendon is reduced back and the retinaculum is repaired.
- **Fig. 8** illustrates this technique and final construct.

PROCEDURAL APPROACH FOR TRIANGULAR FIBROCARTILAGE COMPLEX RECONSTRUCTION

This approach describes an open reconstruction technique for a chronic foveal tear resulting in persistent DRUJ instability with a TFCC that is no longer reparable primarily (Atzei Class 4).[25]

- Inflate the tourniquet.
- Make a longitudinal 4-cm to 5-cm incision between the fifth and sixth extensor compartments, centered over the ulnar head.
- Open the fifth extensor compartment and retract the extensor digiti quinti ulnarly, exposing the DRUJ capsule.
- Create an L-shaped capsulotomy with the longitudinal rim along the dorsal aspect of the sigmoid notch, making a 90-degree turn proximal to the dorsal distal radioulnar ligament toward the ulnar fovea.
- Debride any scar tissue present, and confirm that there is no reparable native TFCC tissue to repair. If there is reasonably reparable tissue, a primary repair may be attempted. Otherwise, a reconstruction as described here should be performed.
- Create a second incision, longitudinally on the volar aspect of the arm from the palmar wrist crease extending 3 to 4 cm proximally between the ulnar neurovascular bundle and the flexor tendons.

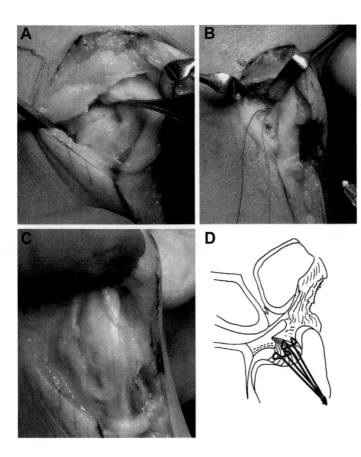

Fig. 8. Operative steps of an open transosseous foveal TFCC repair. (*A*) The radioulnar ligament is incised and retracted. (*B*) Two nonabsorbable sutures are brought from the holes in the fovea to the ulnar cortex of the ulna. (*C*) The TFCC is reduced down to the fovea and sutures are tied on the ulna. (*D*) Illustration of the final construct. (*From* Nakamura T, Sato K, Okazaki M, Toyama Y, Ikegami H. Repair of Foveal Detachment of the Triangular Fibrocartilage Complex: Open and Arthroscopic Transosseous Techniques. Hand Clin. 2011;27(3):281-90; with permission.)

- Multiple graft options may be used; however, here we describe using either the palmaris longus or, if not present, a strip of the flexor carpi ulnaris (FCU).
- On the dorsal aspect of the wrist, the fourth extensor compartment is elevated from the dorsal margin of the sigmoid notch.
- A guidewire is placed through the radius parallel to the articular surface, 1 cm proximal to the joint surface and 5 mm radial to the sigmoid notch.
- This guidewire is overdrilled with a 3.5-mm cannulated drill.
- A second tunnel is created in the ulna at the ulnar neck that ends in the fovea (similar to the tunnel described in the previous section).
- The tendon graft (PL or slip of FCU) is passed through the radial tunnel from dorsal to palmar and one end of the graft is pulled back through the ulnar tunnel.
- The other end of graft is then pulled back through the dorsal incision (proximal to the TFCC and through the palmar capsule).
- Both ends of the graft are then passed through the ulnar tunnel (with one passing volarly and the other passing radially and deep into the ECU sheath).
- The ends of the graft are then tied with the DRUJ compressed with the forearm in neutral rotation. Alternatively, an interference screw may be inserted into the ulnar tunnel following tensioning to eliminate the need for tying the graft.
- **Fig. 9** illustrates this technique and the final construct described.

Tse and colleagues[26] describe the preceding reconstructive technique in an arthroscopic-assisted manner:

- In this technique, the arthroscope is used to assist delivery of the palmaris longus graft.
- After the graft is placed in the radial tunnel, an arthroscopic trochar is introduced into the 4 to 5 portal and exits out the volar capsule between the ulnolunate ligament and short radiolunate ligament to create a window in the volar capsule.
- An arthroscopic grasper is then used to bring the volar limb of the graft into the joint.

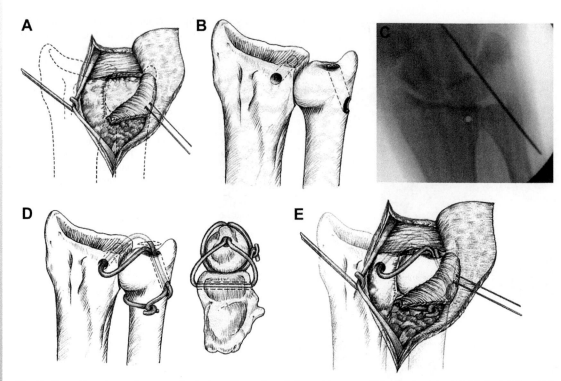

Fig. 9. Operative steps of an open technique for a chronic foveal tear resulting in persistent DRUJ instability with a TFCC that is no longer primarily repairable. (*A*) Surgical exposure through the fifth extensor compartment. (*B*) Illustration depicting radial and ulnar bone tunnels. (*C*) Fluoroscopic image illustrating guidewire assisted ulnar tunnel creation (the radial tunnel is also illustrated). (*D, E*) Illustration of final construct with tendon graft placed. (*From* Adams BD, Berger RA. An anatomic reconstruction of the distal radioulnar ligaments for posttraumatic distal radioulnar joint instability. J Hand Surg Am. 2002;27(2):243-51; with permission.)

- A second grasper through the ulnar tunnel is used to bring the graft back through the ulna.
- The dorsal limb of the graft is placed into the joint through the 4 to 5 portal.
- An arthroscopic grasper is used to retrieve this limb through the ulnar tunnel.
- **Fig. 10** illustrates the arthroscopic assistance technique.

RECOVERY AND REHABILITATION (INCLUDING POSTPROCEDURE CARE)

After arthroscopic **capsular** repairs using the FasT-Fix, patients are immobilized in a simple short arm splint for 2 weeks. Hand therapy for wrist and elbow motion is started at 2 weeks, and strengthening is started at the 4-week mark. Patients are allowed to resume full activity at 6 to 12 weeks.

After arthroscopic **foveal** repairs, patients are placed into a sugar tong splint for 2 weeks and subsequently transitioned to a Munster cast for 4 weeks, allowing for elbow flexion and extension but not forearm pronation or supination. Hand therapy for wrist and elbow motion is started at 6 weeks and strengthening is started at the 8-week mark.

After reconstructive procedures, patients are immobilized in a long-arm splint with the forearm in neutral for 4 weeks. Patients are subsequently transitioned to a short arm splint or cast for 2 more weeks. Patients begin motion at 6 weeks and strengthening exercises at the 8-week mark, and progress to full activity by approximately 4 to 6 months postoperatively.

OUTCOMES

Several treatment options and repair/reconstruction techniques exist. Although few studies exist to directly compare techniques, most have equivalent outcomes.[15–20] In a study comparing clinical outcomes of open versus arthroscopic TFCC repair, Anderson and colleagues[27] noted no difference in clinical outcomes at a mean of 43 months. The investigators did note a 17% total reoperation rate for later DRUJ instability. Abe and colleagues[28] evaluated 24 patients undergoing foveal TFCC tear repairs (8 open, 21 arthroscopic), all using a transosseous tunnel. At a

A

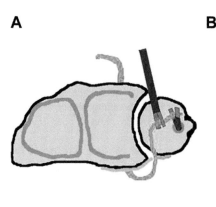

B

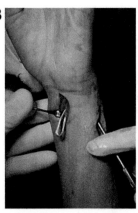

Fig. 10. (*A*, *B*) The volar limb of the palmaris longus graft is placed into the joint with an arthroscopic grasper, and a second grasper is used to bring it back through the ulnar tunnel and the dorsal limb is placed into the joint via the 4 to 5 portal and retrieved similarly through the ulnar tunnel. (*From* Tse WL, Lau SW, Wong WY, Cheng HS, Chow CS, Ho PC, Hung LK. Arthroscopic reconstruction of triangular fibrocartilage complex (TFCC) with tendon graft for chronic DRUJ instability. Injury 2013;44:386-90; with permission.)

mean follow-up of 34 months, the investigators noted no differences in clinical outcomes; however, they did note that the arthroscopic technique took significantly less time. Sarkissian and colleagues[20] evaluated the long-term outcomes of the all-arthroscopic pre-tied suture repair technique in 11 patients with Palmer-type 1B superficial tears (Atzei Class 1). At a mean of 7 years, the investigators reported that grip strength was 98% that of the contralateral wrist, mean wrist flexion and extension was 76° and 73°, respectively, and Quick Disabilities of the Arm, Shoulder, and Hand (QuickDASH) score was 9 (of 100, 0 indicating the least amount of disability and 100 indicating the greatest amount of disability). No surgical-related complications were noted. Park and colleagues[29] evaluated patients with Palmer-type 1B tears who underwent arthroscopic 1-tunnel transosseous foveal repairs. The investigators retrospectively reviewed 16 patients and, at a mean follow-up of 31 months, noted that patients' grip strength, pronosupination arc, visual analog pain score, and QuickDASH improved significantly. They noted no surgery-related complications. Otherwise, there are limited long-term outcome studies evaluating the myriad of treatment techniques for TFCC repair, given the lower incidence and the relatively newer nature and heterogeneity of techniques, indications, and concomitant procedures.

Literature reporting outcomes for reconstructive techniques are also promising. Adams and Berger[25] described their reconstructive technique for instability and outcomes of 14 patients. They reported that stability was restored in 12 of 14 patients with 1-year to 4-year follow-up. All patients achieved near full pronosupination. They noted that 2 patients who did not achieve stability had either a deficient sigmoid notch or an ulnocarpal ligament injury, indicating the importance of preoperative workup, planning,

and surgical indications. Meyer and colleagues[30] reported on 48 patients who underwent reconstruction for instability and noted that stability was achieved in 44 of the 48 patients. They did note, however, that patients reported a loss of approximately 20' of their pronosupination arc. Gillis and colleagues[31] reported the outcomes of 95 consecutive cases treated with the Adams-Berger ligament reconstruction technique for DRUJ instability. At a mean follow-up time of 65 months, the investigators demonstrated that approximately 91% of patients had a stable DRUJ, whereas just more than 3% had some laxity, and just more than 5% were unstable. They described an 86% success rate, with only 12 patients having to undergo an operation for revision. Tse and colleagues[26] reported on the investigators' experience over 10 years using an arthroscopic-assisted TFCC reconstruction for DRUJ instability. With a mean follow-up of 86 months, the investigators noted that 12 of 15 patients were able to return to their jobs. They noted no evidence of DRUJ arthritis and significant improvements in Mayo wrist scores, range of motion, and grip strength.

Although technique differences vary and may continue to be modified, the outcomes of repair and reconstruction are promising when used for appropriate indications.

SUMMARY

The recognition and treatment of TFCC injuries are nuanced and require a discerning and technically proficient surgeon. An understanding of concomitant injuries, as well as the pathophysiology of TFCC injuries, helps guide treatment. Multiple techniques demonstrate success in improving pain and restoring function with the technique selection guided by patient, injury, and surgeon factors.

CLINICS CARE POINTS

- A thorough understanding of the anatomy, pathophysiology, and the patient's physical examination and goals helps ensure appropriate treatment/technique selection.

- DRUJ instability should be treated early with a foveal TFCC repair.

- In the absence of DRUJ instability, a period of 4 weeks of immobilization should be attempted as initial treatment.

- Preoperative imaging (MRI, MRI arthrogram) is very helpful in identifying the severity and location of the tear, thereby dictating which type of treatment is necessary.

- Chronicity of the injury is not as important as the quality of the tissue when considering TFCC repair or reconstruction.

- Superficial skin incisions with blunt dissection down to and through the wrist capsule are important to prevent injury to sensory nerve branches and tendons during arthroscopy.

- The technique for TFCC repair or reconstruction should be dependent on the quality of the tissue and the surgeon's comfort level with any particular technique.

DISCLOSURE

The authors have no relevant disclosures pertaining to the production of this article. The content of this work is solely the responsibility of the authors. No authors have any conflicts of interest related to this work and no benefits in any form have been received or will be received related directly or indirectly to the subject of this article.

REFERENCES

1. Kleinman WB. Stability of the distal radioulna joint: biomechanics, pathophysiology, physical diagnosis, and restoration of function what we have learned in 25 years. J Hand Surg Am 2007;32(7):1086–106.

2. Nakamura T, Yabe Y. Histological anatomy of the triangular fibrocartilage complex of the human wrist. Ann Anat 2000;182(6):567–72.

3. Sasao S, Beppu M, Kihara H, et al. An anatomical study of the ligaments of the ulnar compartment of the wrist. Hand Surg 2003;8(2):219–26.

4. Schmidt H-M. [The anatomy of the ulnocarpal complex]. Orthopade 2004;33(6):628–37.

5. Yan B, Xu Z, Chen Y, et al. Prevalence of triangular fibrocartilage complex injuries in patients with distal radius fractures: a 3.0T magnetic resonance imaging study. J Int Med Res 2019;47(8):3648–55.

6. Baratz ME. Central TFCC tears in baseball players. Hand Clin 2012;28(3):339.

7. Howard TC. Elite athlete: chronic DRUJ instability or central TFC tears. Hand Clin 2012;28(3):341–2.

8. Palmer AK, Werner FW. The triangular fibrocartilage complex of the wrist–anatomy and function. J Hand Surg Am 1981;6(2):153–62.

9. Bednar MS, Arnoczky SP, Weiland AJ. The microvasculature of the triangular fibrocartilage complex: its clinical significance. J Hand Surg Am 1991;16(6):1101–5.

10. Thiru RG, Ferlic DC, Clayton ML, et al. Arterial anatomy of the triangular fibrocartilage of the wrist and its surgical significance. J Hand Surg Am 1986;11(2):258–63.

11. Palmer AK. Triangular fibrocartilage complex lesions: a classification. J Hand Surg Am 1989;14(4):594–606.

12. Atzei A, Luchetti R. Foveal TFCC tear classification and treatment. Hand Clin 2011;27(3):263–72.

13. Pang EQ, Yao J. Ulnar-sided wrist pain in the athlete (TFCC/DRUJ/ECU). Curr Rev Musculoskelet Med 2017;10(1):53–61.

14. Park MJ, Jagadish A, Yao J. The rate of triangular fibrocartilage injuries requiring surgical intervention. Orthopedics 2010;33(11):806.

15. Yao J. All-arthroscopic repair of peripheral triangular fibrocartilage complex tears using FasT-Fix. Hand Clin 2011;27(3):237–42.

16. Pederzini LA, Tosi M, Prandini M, et al. All-inside suture technique for Palmer class 1B triangular fibrocartilage repair. Arthroscopy 2007;23(10):1130.e1–4.

17. Whipple TL, Geissler WB. Arthroscopic management of wrist triangular fibrocartilage complex injuries in the athlete. Orthopedics 1993;16(9):1061–7.

18. Estrella EP, Hung L-K, Ho P-C, et al. Arthroscopic repair of triangular fibrocartilage complex tears. Arthroscopy 2007;23(7):729–37, 737.e1.

19. Corso SJ, Savoie FH, Geissler WB, et al. Arthroscopic repair of peripheral avulsions of the triangular fibrocartilage complex of the wrist: a multicenter study. Arthroscopy 1997;13(1):78–84.

20. Sarkissian EJ, Burn MB, Yao J. Long-term outcomes of all-arthroscopic pre-tied suture device triangular fibrocartilage complex repair. J Wrist Surg 2019;8(5):403–7.

21. Papapetropoulos PA, Ruch DS. Repair of arthroscopic triangular fibrocartilage complex tears in athletes. Hand Clin 2009;25(3):389–94.

22. Park Y. All-arthroscopic knotless suture anchor repair of triangular fibrocartilage complex fovea tear by the 2-portal technique. Arthrosc Tech 2014;3(6):e673–7.

23. Nakamura T, Sato K, Okazaki M, et al. Repair of foveal detachment of the triangular fibrocartilage

complex: open and arthroscopic transosseous techniques. Hand Clin 2011;27(3):281–90.

24. Atzei A, Luchetti R, Braidotti F. Arthroscopic foveal repair of the triangular fibrocartilage complex. J Wrist Surg 2015;04(01):022–30.

25. Adams BD, Berger RA. An anatomic reconstruction of the distal radioulnar ligaments for posttraumatic distal radioulnar joint instability. J Hand Surg Am 2002;27(2):243–51.

26. Tse WL, Lau SW, Wong WY, et al. Arthroscopic reconstruction of triangular fibrocartilage complex (TFCC) with tendon graft for chronic DRUJ instability. Injury 2013;44:386–90.

27. Anderson ML, Larson AN, Moran SL, et al. Clinical comparison of arthroscopic versus open repair of triangular fibrocartilage complex tears. J Hand Surg 2008;33(5):675–82.

28. Abe Y, Fujii K, Fujisawa T. Midterm results after open versus arthroscopic transosseous repair for foveal tears of the triangular fibrocartilage complex. J Wrist Surg 2018;7(4):292–7.

29. Park JH, Kim D, Park JW. Arthroscopic one-tunnel transosseous foveal repair for triangular fibrocartilage complex (TFCC) peripheral tear. Arch Orthop Trauma Surg 2018;138(1):131–8.

30. Meyer D, Schweizer A, Nagy L. Anatomic reconstruction of distal radioulnar ligaments with tendon graft for treating distal radioulnar joint instability: surgical technique and outcome. Tech Hand Up Extrem Surg 2017;21(3):107–13.

31. Gillis JA, Soreide E, Khouri JS, et al. Outcomes of the Adams–Berger ligament reconstruction for the distal radioulnar joint instability in 95 consecutive cases. J Wrist Surg 2019;8(4):268–75.

Failed Triangular Fibrocartilage Complex Repair and Reconstruction

Remy V. Rabinovich, MD[a,*], David S. Zelouf, MD[b]

KEYWORDS

- Failed TFCC • Revision wrist arthroscopy • Ulnar-sided wrist pain • DRUJ

KEY POINTS

- Failed triangular fibrocartilage complex surgery is complex, emanating from multiple factors, both patient and surgeon-related.
- Surgical candidate selection is critical and requires full assessment of the patient's psychosocial status and involvement in any litigation or worker's compensation claims.
- Surgeon-related causes, such as misdiagnosis, postoperative complications, and intraoperative technical errors, should be minimized with complete patient evaluation and careful preventive treatment strategies.

INTRODUCTION

Pathology involving the ulnar side of the wrist, notoriously known as the "black box," has always been a challenge to accurately diagnose and treat. One of the more common sources of pain in this region is the triangular fibrocartilage complex (TFCC). This particular structure's intricate anatomy and restricted vascular supply, along with constant axial and torsional stresses, make it prone to frequent injury with limited ability to heal.[1] Treatment of TFCC injury can be classified as acute or chronic, and when conservative management is unsuccessful, it can be approached surgically, either open, arthroscopic, or a combination of both.[2] Most reports on surgical outcomes following open and arthroscopic TFCC repair primarily consist of small, retrospective case series with midterm follow-up. Acceptable functional results have been demonstrated, with mean postoperative outcome scores ranging from 7.7 to 36 and 70 to 94 on the Disabilities of the Arm, Shoulder, and Hand (DASH) and Modified Mayo Wrist Score (MMWS) tools, respectively.[3–10] Mean postoperative grip strength has ranged from 75% to 98% of the contralateral side[6,8,10,11] with mean postoperative visual analog scale (VAS) pain scores of either 0 or 1.[3,4,12] When comparing open versus arthroscopic techniques, both groups demonstrate improvements in DASH, MMWS, and VAS scores as well as grip strength. No significant differences in clinical outcomes have been identified between the 2 approaches.[3,8]

Although TFCC repair and reconstruction have been associated with generally positive postoperative outcomes, complications and failed TFCC surgery are not infrequent. A myriad of complications have been described, and include injury to the dorsal sensory branch of the ulnar nerve (DSBUN), persistent pain, distal radioulnar joint (DRUJ) instability, and suture irritation potentially requiring reoperation. The definition of failed TFCC surgery, and surgery in general, is, however, ill defined. It can be related to numerous factors, both patient and surgeon-related. In this review, we aim to (1) better define failed surgery,

Conflict of Interest: The authors have nothing to disclose.
^a New York Hand and Wrist Center – Northwell Health, 210 East 64th Street, 5th Floor, New York, NY 10065, USA; ^b Philadelphia Hand to Shoulder Center and Thomas Jefferson University Hospitals, 834 Chestnut Street, Suite G-114, Philadelphia, PA 19107, USA
* Corresponding author.
E-mail address: remyrabinovich@gmail.com

hand.theclinics.com

particularly related to the surgical management of TFCC injury, and (2) analyze the etiology of unsuccessful TFCC repair and reconstruction as well as revision treatment strategies.

NATURE OF THE PROBLEM: DEFINING FAILED TRIANGULAR FIBROCARTILAGE COMPLEX SURGERY

The difficulty in managing failed TFCC repair or reconstruction emanates from the ambiguity in defining failure. Failed surgery can be defined as no meaningful improvement in one's symptoms at final postoperative follow-up. Part of the complexity is that the notion of failed surgery stems from multiple facets, both patient and surgeon-related. Patient-related factors contributing to failure can be subjective or objective. Subjective variables include postoperative symptoms (eg, pain, feeling of weakness) and the inability to return to work, sport, or routine activities of daily living. These subjective variables can be difficult to elucidate, as they can be confounded by both internal (eg, anxiety, depression, malingering, Munchausen) and external (eg, litigation, workers' compensation) components and motives. Objective factors include measured weakness (such as that obtained through grip strength measurements), stiffness, and instability. Surgeon-related factors contributing to failure include improper diagnosis and surgical complications, as well as technical inadequacies or insufficiencies. The interpretation of a surgical complication is variable and benchmarking data are lacking to definitively establish which intraoperative or postoperative event should be considered a complication.[13]

In relation to TFCC repair or reconstruction, failed surgery can stem from 4 main etiologies. The first is improper patient selection; specifically, patients with psychosocial problems or those involved in litigation disputes.[13–16] The second is improper diagnosis. Symptoms at the ulnar side of the wrist present a diagnostic challenge due to the complex anatomy in this region and, therefore, not all symptoms at the ulnar wrist are secondary to TFCC pathology. The last 2 are complications following surgery and intraoperative technical inadequacies or insufficiencies.

ETIOLOGY OF FAILED TRIANGULAR FIBROCARTILAGE COMPLEX SURGERY AND TREATMENT STRATEGIES
Improper Patient Selection

An unsuccessful trial of nonoperative management for treating a TFCC tear does not necessarily warrant surgical management. Proper patient selection is paramount following evaluation of the patient's psychosocial status and involvement in any litigation or workers' compensation claims. Although no direct correlation has been established between these factors and failed TFCC repair or reconstruction, other upper extremity procedures have been linked to worse outcomes among patients with these issues. Depression has been recognized as a predictor of disability and pain intensity among patients undergoing minor hand surgery procedures (ie, carpal tunnel release, trigger finger release, benign soft tissue mass excision) in addition to being associated with higher DASH scores among patients treated for carpal tunnel syndrome, de Quervain tendinitis, lateral elbow pain, trigger finger, and distal radius fracture.[17,18] Increasing levels of patient anxiety and pain interference have also been correlated with lower patient-reported upper extremity function.[16,18] Litigation involvement, including workers' compensation, has also been associated with diminished postoperative outcomes after hand surgery. Workers' compensation status has been linked to higher recurrence rates and poorer patient-reported outcomes following primary carpal tunnel release,[19,20] in addition to being a predictor of postoperative pain following revision carpal tunnel surgery.[21] Rohman and colleagues[22] have also shown workers' compensation to be a risk factor for surgical failure of scapholunate ligament repair and reconstruction among 82 wrists with a median of 150 days of follow-up.

Proper patient selection entails a high index of suspicion for identifying patients with potential litigation involvement and/or psychosocial issues. The latter may be best cared for using a multidisciplinary approach to help diagnose and treat these issues alongside treatment of the TFCC injury. Screening tools, such as QuickDASH measurements and review of systems checklists, can help identify patients with signs and symptoms of depression, anxiety, and conversion disorder, as well as catastrophizing and/or malingering behaviors. Factitious disorders of the hand can be categorized into 4 groups: factitious wound creation/manipulation, factitious edema, psychopathological dystonia, and psychopathological complex regional pain syndrome. Each is associated with its own unique characteristics based on patient presentation, utilization of medical resources, return-to-work rate, and education level.[23]

Misdiagnosis

Accurate diagnosis and proper treatment of ulnar-sided wrist pathology can be one of the most challenging tasks for even the most experienced hand surgeon. A seemingly endless list of confounders and differential diagnoses can potentially mask the true pathology and make an accurate diagnosis difficult. The patient's history of present illness may contribute important diagnostic clues. A description of the mechanism of injury as well as any work, hobby, or sport-related repetitive movements can be vital, as TFCC and DRUJ injury are often associated with hyperpronation and axial loading forces. Physical examination also plays a pivotal role in assessing the TFCC and its neighboring structures, such as the flexor and extensor carpi ulnaris and extensor digitorum communis tendons, and the ulnocarpal, distal radioulnar, and pisotriquetral joints, as well as the ulnar extrinsic and intrinsic ligaments. Diagnostic imaging plays a key role in the workup. Radiographs provide a visualization of pertinent anatomy, including ulnar variance, joint space/cartilage loss, and overall alignment. They also show the presence of a preexisting or acute fracture, dislocation, deformity, intraosseous lesion, or arthritis. Live fluoroscopy can provide a dynamic assessment of osseous and ligamentous structures, including their role in maintaining joint stability. Ultrasound can pinpoint vascular, bony, or soft tissue lesions, and can also help illustrate the status of adjacent nerves or tendons. MRI, with or without arthrography, has become a powerful tool in assessing the wrist. The sensitivity and specificity for the diagnosis of central and peripheral TFCC tears using MR arthrography is 84% to 95% and 95% to 100%, respectively.[24,25] When stratified, the diagnosis of peripheral tears is less accurate using this modality, with a sensitivity of 85% and specificity of 76%.[26] Diagnostic conventional arthrography and computed tomography (CT) have also been extensively used; CT in particular has been found useful in depicting pathology in the DRUJ. Although invasive, the gold standard in assessing intra-articular wrist pathology is arthroscopy, which reveals more lesions than any other imaging modality.[27,28]

Failure to recognize concomitant pathology often associated with TFCC tears can lead to continued postoperative pain and/or instability. Jang and colleagues[29] reported their outcomes of revision wrist arthroscopy and noted that on second look following index TFCC debridement or repair, a missed diagnosis of DRUJ instability, dynamic ulnar impaction, and dynamic scapholunate interosseous ligament (SLIL) instability were present. Dynamic ulnar impaction was addressed with a Feldon arthroscopic wafer procedure. Dynamic SLIL instability was treated with thermal shrinkage of the SLIL ± Kirschner-wire fixation,

and DRUJ instability was treated with outside-in peripheral TFCC reattachment and retensioning. All groups consisted of a minimum of 4 weeks of postoperative splinting plus hand therapy, and significant improvements in VAS pain scores were noted at final follow-up. Misdiagnosis and failure to treat TFCC tears along with concomitant ulnar-sided wrist pathology was also reported by Tomori and colleagues.[30] The investigators reported the case of a college hockey player whose symptoms failed to improve following surgical stabilization of recurrent extensor carpi ulnaris (ECU) subluxation until the patient's concomitant TFCC tear was diagnosed and repaired. Lourie and his group[31] analyzed the presentation and treatment of triquetrohamate (TH) impaction syndrome (THIS), highlighting that almost half of the patients in their series were initially misdiagnosed with having a TFCC tear. The investigators highlighted the importance of obtaining postero-anterior (PA) plus radial and ulnar deviation radiographs in addition to CT or MRI to better define TH pathology. Fifty percent of patients responded to initial conservative treatment, whereas 78% of patients who underwent surgery noted complete relief of their symptoms and returned to preinjury activity levels. Three patients had arthroscopic debridement of the joint and/or microfracture, and 6 patients underwent open partial excision of either the hamate or triquetrum. The remainder of patients who were treated surgically had mild pain with preinjury activities and were overall satisfied with their results. Along with THIS, an underreported and often misdiagnosed clinical entity leading to failed TFCC surgery is radial shaft and distal radius malunion. These conditions alter normal DRUJ kinematics even when the TFCC is intact. In biomechanical studies, as dorsal angulation and translation deformity of the distal radius increase, TFCC strain is increased and significant volar and distal displacement of the ulnar head ensues; this effect is heightened with forearm supination.[32–34] Malunited radial shaft fractures, often seen in patients with a history of trauma before skeletal maturity, can present with supination dissociation characterized by volar DRUJ instability with supination, persistent ulnar-sided wrist pain, and restricted pronosupination.[35] These patients can present having previously failed soft tissue reconstruction and so obtaining forearm radiographs during initial evaluation is critical to not miss the diagnosis of malunion. Corrective radial shaft osteotomy alone can help restore pain-free DRUJ stability and function.[36] **Fig. 1**A and B show an apex volar radial shaft malunion in a 25-year-old man who was treated with closed reduction and cast immobilization for his right radius fracture that was sustained

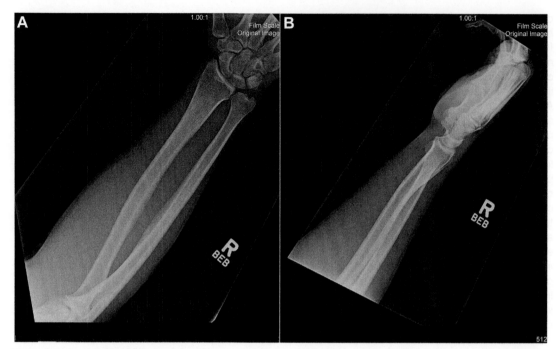

Fig. 1. (A) PA radiograph of the right forearm depicting evidence of a healed distal one-third radial shaft fracture. (B) Lateral radiograph of the same forearm, better depicting evidence of a healed, malunited, apex volar distal one-third radial shaft fracture.

10 years prior. He presented to our office with ulnar-sided wrist pain, volar DRUJ instability (**Fig. 2**), and failed arthroscopic TFCC repair 5 years prior. After undergoing a corrective opening wedge osteotomy of his radius, the patient reported minimal discomfort and exhibited a stable DRUJ with excellent range of motion (ROM) and consolidation at the osteotomy site at final follow-up (**Fig. 3**A and B).

Surgical Complications

Several notable complications following surgical repair or reconstruction of the TFCC have been reported. Whether performed open or arthroscopically, irritation of the DSBUN or neuroma formation has been noted in up to 36% of patients, without a significant difference between approaches.[8,37] This is often related to 6R and 6U portal placement during arthroscopy or during retractor positioning when the TFCC is treated through an open approach. Identifying and protecting the nerve along with careful retractor placement can help prevent injury, along with avoidance of using the 6U portal as a working portal. Transient neurapraxia, mainly at the finger level, has also been reported, typically as a result of finger traction.[38] Caution is advised during surgical set up of the traction tower and finger traps. Soft tissue irritation from prominent suture knots

following TFCC repair is not uncommon.[8,37] Proper suture tying, cutting the suture tails flush with the knot, and allowing for adequate soft tissue coverage can help minimize irritation. All-arthroscopic and knotless suture techniques also can help reduce morbidity, although limited outcome data have been reported.[39,40] As with most intra-articular wrist injuries, stiffness following TFCC surgery can be seen. In a retrospective review of more than 10,000 wrist arthroscopies, for various wrist pathologies, 30 cases of stiffness were reported to be directly related to the procedure.[40] Preventive strategies to decrease stiffness include avoiding prolonged immobilization following TFCC debridement and limiting it to no more than 4 to 6 weeks after repair, while allowing elbow flexion and extension. Early use of hand therapy is also recommended, particularly in those patients with early-identified stiffness. Less common but known complications include infection, iatrogenic cartilage, and ligament and/ or tendon injury. Infection following arthroscopic wrist surgery is rare, with only 2 reported cases among more than 500 consecutive wrist arthroscopies in a study by Hoel and colleagues,[41] both of which involved the placement of percutaneous pins. Iatrogenic cartilage, ligament, and/or tendon damage can occur as well. These events can be minimized with proper portal position, deliberate

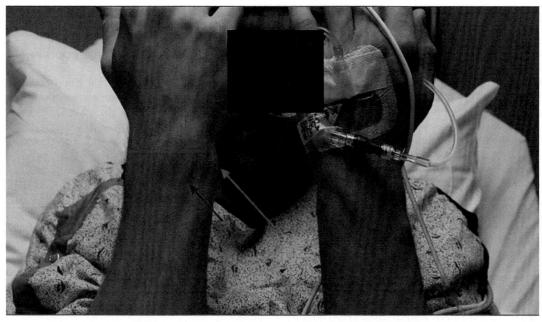

Fig. 2. Clinical photograph of our patient showing the dorsal ulnar sulcus sign (*short blue arrow*), characteristic of volar subluxation of the distal ulna (*long red arrow*) during supination of the right wrist.

and nonforceful insertion of instruments, and careful use of electrothermal devices with the presence of outflow to prevent chondrolysis.

Technical Considerations

Although complications mostly comprise the novel issues seen postoperatively, persistent or worsening preoperative symptoms, in particular pain and instability, can continue after TFCC surgery. These are more likely related to inadequate or insufficient technical performance by the surgeon. Incorrectly or incompletely performing the planned surgical procedure may result in surgical failure. Examples include inadequate or insufficient debridement of a central TFCC tear or failing

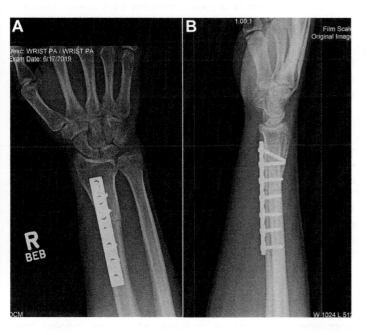

Fig. 3. (*A*) PA radiograph and (*B*) lateral radiograph of our patient's right wrist, 3 months after undergoing a volar, opening wedge radius osteotomy, stabilized with a 7-hole 3.5-mm stainless steel dynamic compression plate.

to repair a nondestabilizing peripheral tear back down to capsule. Insufficient or inadequate arthroscopic assessment of the TFCC (failure to fully visualize the tear or evaluate and diagnose a foveal disruption of the ligamentum subcruentum) can lead to persistent DRUJ instability and continued pain. Continued ulnar-sided wrist pain following arthroscopic debridement of stable, central TFCC tears with or without debridement of stable lunotriquetrial (LT) tears can be effectively managed with ulnar shortening osteotomy. Hulsizer and colleagues[42] reported complete pain relief and return to full and usual work in 12 of 13 patients (average ulnar variance of 0.4 mm) who underwent an ulnar shortening osteotomy of at least 2 mm after failing arthroscopic debridement of isolated stable, central TFCC tears with or without debridement of a concomitant, stable LT tear. As highlighted previously, failure to address concomitant pathology (ie, LT or scapholunate ligament [SL] tears, ECU tendinosis/instability, ulnocarpal impaction) can lead to failed TFCC surgery as well. This can be minimized with adequate radiocarpal and midcarpal arthroscopic assessment of the wrist. As with most surgical procedures, surgeon experience plays a pivotal role. Leclercq and colleagues[38] demonstrated a learning curve with wrist arthroscopy and that both a regular practice of the technique (>25 wrist arthroscopies per year) and the number of years of experience (more than 5 years) significantly decreased the rate of complications.

TREATMENT

The treatment of failed TFCC repair or reconstructions is diverse and depends on numerous factors. Unsatisfactory results in patients with psychosocial issues or those involved in litigation or workers' compensation claims should be approached with caution. Conservative measures should almost always be considered first unless a clear mechanical problem exists that has not been properly addressed. Even then, the results of reoperation in this patient population can be unpredictable at best. Literature acknowledging an association between this subset of patients and the results of reoperation after failed TFCC surgery is lacking. Patients with psychological issues such as schizophrenia and depression have, however, been shown to have greater postoperative issues necessitating emergency room visits following elective outpatient hand surgery.[43] Depression along with patient involvement in workers' compensation claims have each been identified to be predictors of poorer postoperative outcomes following various hand surgery procedures,

including revision carpal tunnel release.[16–21] Taking these correlations into consideration, reoperation after failed TFCC surgery should be approached hesitantly in this subgroup of patients, as they can portend diminished outcomes.

Failed TFCC repair or reconstruction due to a missed diagnosis of a concomitant or completely unrelated pathology entails treatment of the root problem. This often involves revision surgery and, subsequently, improved results can be anticipated. Jang and colleagues[29] demonstrated improved VAS pain scores after seemingly isolated and appropriately managed type 1A and 1C TFCC tears were secondarily treated with repeat wrist arthroscopy and stabilization of initially missed dynamic ulnar impaction or SLIL instability. Similarly, Tomori and colleagues[30] noted definitive resolution of symptoms and return to competitive-level performance after a concomitant TFCC tear was missed and subsequently repaired in an ice hockey player initially treated for isolated ECU instability.

Management of surgical complications following TFCC repair or reconstruction is complex. Treatment strategies should be individualized based on the specific type of complication and the degree to which the patient is affected by it. Complications such as stiffness and neurapraxia should initially be approached nonoperatively with hand therapy, as they often respond to conservative measures. Preventive strategies for wrist stiffness include immobilization for no more than 6 weeks following TFCC repair, as well as early digital ROM and limb elevation to decrease edema. If these measures have been exhausted for at least 3 months postoperatively, arthrolysis and capsular release can be considered, as this has been shown to improve ROM and grip strength.[44] Persistent neurapraxia and/or nerve pain postoperatively may suggest the presence of a neuroma. Neuroma formation in the setting of TFCC surgery most commonly involves the DSBUN, and preventive strategies include caution when exposing the ulnar side of the wrist and using the safe zone for establishing the 6R portal, which is found within the proximal fifth (19%) of a line drawn from the ulnar styloid to the fourth dorsal web space.[45] Conservative options should be maximized before considering surgical intervention, especially in patients who are averse to or cannot tolerate surgery. These include various physical therapy modalities, desensitization protocols, analgesic and neuropathic agents, and corticosteroid injections.[46] Surgical management of neuromas involving cutaneous branches of the median, radial, and ulnar nerves around the wrist includes a multitude of options ranging from neuroma resection with or without nerve repair/reconstruction or transposition into muscle or vein. Results are mixed and unpredictable.[47–49] Treatment of less common complications, such as infection and tendon and ligament injuries, should be individualized. Superficial wound infections often respond to a regimen of antibiotic therapy, whereas deep infections may require surgical irrigation and debridement in addition to antibiotics. Inadvertent tendon and ligament injuries often require repair, especially if instability ensues or the patient's function is compromised as a result.

If a patient's symptoms persist following TFCC repair and it is clear that legitimate ongoing unaddressed pathology is present, revision wrist arthroscopy and TFCC stabilization may be warranted, which can lead to clinically meaningful improvement. Inadequate or insufficient debridement of a central TFCC tear or failure to repair a nondestabilizing peripheral tear back down to capsule during the index surgery warrants a reoperation to definitively address the underlying problem. Insufficient or inadequate arthroscopic assessment of the TFCC without identifying a foveal disruption of the ligamentum subcruentum can lead to persistent DRUJ instability and continued pain. This requires revision surgery and stabilization of the deep radioulnar fibers of the TFCC to the fovea.[4] In this setting, if the distal radioulnar ligaments are incompetent, a reconstruction with a tendon graft may be necessary.[50] As mentioned earlier, complete radiocarpal and midcarpal arthroscopic assessment of the wrist, with or without arthroscopic assessment of the DRUJ, depending on other related findings, is key to minimize inadequate or insufficient treatment of TFCC pathology.

SUMMARY

The evaluation and treatment of TFCC tears is faced with multiple challenges and can result in unsuccessful repair or reconstruction. Failed TFCC surgery can be defined as no meaningful improvement in one's symptoms at final postoperative follow-up and can stem from multiple facets, both patient and surgeon-related. Patient-related factors can be objective or subjective, at times confounded by external or internal motives. Thus, proper selection of surgical candidates is pivotal, requiring full assessment and a high index of suspicion for identifying patients with potential litigation involvement and psychosocial issues. These variables are associated with poorer outcomes, and a multidisciplinary approach is often warranted. Surgeon-related causes of failed TFCC surgery include improper diagnosis, surgical complications, and technical inadequacies or insufficiencies. The proper diagnosis of TFCC injury along with any potential concomitant or confounding wrist pathology can be a challenging task for even the most experienced hand surgeon. Complete evaluation includes a pertinent history, physical examination, and selection of imaging that allows for an adequate static and dynamic assessment of the TFCC and its neighboring structures. Common surgical complications following TFCC surgery include DSBUN injury, soft tissue irritation from prominent sutures, and stiffness, whereas less common complications are infection and iatrogenic injury to cartilage, ligaments, or tendons. These events can be minimized with proper attention and awareness of their potential as well as the implementation of careful preventive strategies both intraoperatively and perioperatively. Technical inadequacies and insufficiencies during surgery can lead to persistent symptoms postoperatively. Making sure to adequately and sufficiently address TFCC injury in addition to any concomitant pathology is critical to optimize clinical outcome. In carefully selected patients, revision surgery can be successful, particularly if the index procedure did not completely address the relevant pathology.

CLINICS CARE POINTS

- Failed TFCC surgery is complex, emanating from multiple factors, both patient and surgeon-related.
- Surgical candidate selection is critical and requires full assessment of the patient's psychosocial status and involvement in any litigation or workers' compensation claims.
- Surgeon-related causes, such as misdiagnosis, postoperative complications, and intraoperative technical errors, should be minimized with complete patient evaluation and careful preventive treatment strategies.

REFERENCES

1. Bednar MS, Arnoczky SP, Weiland AJ. The microvasculature of the triangular fibrocartilage complex: its clinical significance. J Hand Surg Am 1991;16(6):1101–5.

2. Palmer AK. Triangular fibrocartilage complex lesions: a classification. J Hand Surg Am 1989;14(4):594–606.

3. Luchetti R, Atzei A, Cozzolino R, et al. Comparison between open and arthroscopic-assisted foveal triangular fibrocartilage complex repair for post-traumatic distal radio-ulnar joint instability. J Hand Surg Eur 2014;39(8):845–55.

4. Atzei A, Luchetti R, Braidotti F. Arthroscopic foveal repair of the triangular fibrocartilage complex. J Wrist Surg 2015;4(1):22–30.

5. Iwasaki N, Nishida K, Motomiya M, et al. Arthroscopic-assisted repair of avulsed triangular fibrocartilage complex to the fovea of the ulnar head: a 2- to 4-year follow-up study. Arthroscopy 2011;27(10):1371–8.

6. Shinohara T, Tatebe M, Okui N, et al. Arthroscopically assisted repair of triangular fibrocartilage complex foveal tears. J Hand Surg Am 2013;38(2):271–7.

7. Cooney WP, Linscheid RL, Dobyns JH. Triangular fibrocartilage tears. J Hand Surg Am 1994;19(1):143–54.

8. Anderson ML, Larson AN, Moran SL, et al. Clinical comparison of arthroscopic versus open repair of triangular fibrocartilage complex tears. J Hand Surg Am 2008;33(5):675–82.

9. Ruch DS, Papadonikolakis A. Arthroscopically assisted repair of peripheral triangular fibrocartilage complex tears: factors affecting outcome. Arthroscopy 2005;21(9):1126–30.

10. Chou KH, Sarris IK, Sotereanos DG. Suture anchor repair of ulnar-sided triangular fibrocartilage complex tears. J Hand Surg Br 2003;28(6):546–50.

11. Trumble TE, Gilbert M, Vedder N. Isolated tears of the triangular fibrocartilage: management by early arthroscopic repair. J Hand Surg Am 1997;22(1):57–65.

12. Selles CA, d'Ailly PN, Schep NWL. Patient-reported outcomes following arthroscopic triangular fibrocartilage complex repair. J Wrist Surg 2020;9(1):58–62.

13. Visser A, Ubbink DT, Gouma DJ, et al. Which clinical scenarios do surgeons record as complications? A benchmarking study of seven hospitals. BMJ Open 2015;5(6):e007500.

14. Moskal MJ, Savoie FH, Field LD. Arthroscopic capsulodesis of the lunotriquetral joint. Clin Sports Med 2001;20(1):141–53. ix-x.

15. Gire J, Alokozai A, Sheikholeslami N, et al. Maximization personality, disability and symptoms of psychosocial disease in hand surgery patients. J Surg Orthop Adv 2020;29(2):106–11.

16. Kazmers NH, Hung M, Rane AA, et al. Association of physical function, anxiety, and pain interference in nonshoulder upper extremity patients using the PROMIS platform. J Hand Surg Am 2017;42(10):781–7.

17. Vranceanu AM, Jupiter JB, Mudgal CS, et al. Predictors of pain intensity and disability after minor hand surgery. J Hand Surg Am 2010;35(6):956–60.

18. Ring D, Kadzielski J, Fabian L, et al. Self-reported upper extremity health status correlates with depression. J Bone Joint Surg Am 2006;88(9):1983–8.

19. Strasberg SR, Novak CB, Mackinnon SE, et al. Subjective and employment outcome following secondary carpal tunnel surgery. Ann Plast Surg 1994;32(5):485–9.

20. Cotton P. Symptoms may return after carpal tunnel surgery. JAMA 1991;265(15):1922, 5.

21. Zieske L, Ebersole GC, Davidge K, et al. Revision carpal tunnel surgery: a 10-year review of intraoperative findings and outcomes. J Hand Surg Am 2013;38(8):1530–9.

22. Rohman EM, Agel J, Putnam MD, et al. Scapholunate interosseous ligament injuries: a retrospective review of treatment and outcomes in 82 wrists. J Hand Surg Am 2014;39(10):2020–6.

23. O'Connor EA, Grunert BK, Matloub HS, et al. Factitious hand disorders: review of 29 years of multidisciplinary care. J Hand Surg Am 2013;38(8):1590–8.

24. Petsatodis E, Pilavaki M, Kalogera A, et al. Comparison between conventional MRI and MR arthrography in the diagnosis of triangular fibrocartilage tears and correlation with arthroscopic findings. Injury 2019;50(8):1464–9.

25. Smith TO, Drew B, Toms AP, et al. Diagnostic accuracy of magnetic resonance imaging and magnetic resonance arthrography for triangular fibrocartilaginous complex injury: a systematic review and meta-analysis. J Bone Joint Surg Am 2012;94(9):824–32.

26. Rüegger C, Schmid MR, Pfirrmann CW, et al. Peripheral tear of the triangular fibrocartilage: depiction with MR arthrography of the distal radioulnar joint. AJR Am J Roentgenol 2007;188(1):187–92.

27. Tanaka T, Yoshioka H, Ueno T, et al. Comparison between high-resolution MRI with a microscopy coil and arthroscopy in triangular fibrocartilage complex injury. J Hand Surg Am 2006;31(8):1308–14.

28. Chung KC, Zimmerman NB, Travis MT. Wrist arthrography versus arthroscopy: a comparative study of 150 cases. J Hand Surg Am 1996;21(4):591–4.

29. Jang E, Danoff JR, Rajfer RA, et al. Revision wrist arthroscopy after failed primary arthroscopic treatment. J Wrist Surg 2014;3(1):30–6.

30. Tomori Y, Nanno M, Takai S. Recurrent dislocation of the extensor carpi ulnaris tendon with ulnar-sided triangular fibrocartilage complex injury in an ice hockey player: a case report. J Nippon Med Sch 2020.

31. Lourie GM, Booth C, Nathan R. Triquetrohamate impaction syndrome: an unrecognized cause of ulnar-sided wrist pain; its presentation further defined. Hand (N Y) 2017;12(4):382–8.

32. Adams BD. Effects of radial deformity on distal radioulnar joint mechanics. J Hand Surg Am 1993; 18(3):492–8.

33. Nishiwaki M, Welsh M, Gammon B, et al. Volar subluxation of the ulnar head in dorsal translation deformities of distal radius fractures: an in vitro biomechanical study. J Orthop Trauma 2015;29(6): 295–300.

34. Nishiwaki M, Welsh M, Gammon B, et al. Distal radioulnar joint kinematics in simulated dorsally angulated distal radius fractures. J Hand Surg Am 2014; 39(4):656–63.

35. Oda T, Wada T, Isogai S, et al. Corrective osteotomy for volar instability of the distal radioulnar joint associated with radial shaft malunion. J Hand Surg Eur Vol 2007;32(5):573–7.

36. Miller A, Lightdale-Miric N, Eismann E, et al. Outcomes of isolated radial osteotomy for volar distal radioulnar joint instability following radial malunion in children. J Hand Surg Am 2018;43(1):81.e1–8.

37. Dunn JC, Polmear MM, Nesti LJ. Surgical repair of acute TFCC injury. Hand (N Y) 2019;15(5):674–8.

38. Leclercq C, Mathoulin C, Mo EWAS. Complications of wrist arthroscopy: a multicenter study based on 10,107 arthroscopies. J Wrist Surg 2016;5(4):320–6.

39. Yao J, Lee AT. All-arthroscopic repair of Palmer 1B triangular fibrocartilage complex tears using the FasT-Fix device. J Hand Surg Am 2011;36(5): 836–42.

40. Geissler WB. Arthroscopic knotless peripheral ulnar-sided TFCC repair. J Wrist Surg 2015;4(2):143–7.

41. Hoel RJ, Mittelsteadt MJ, Samborski SA, et al. Preoperative antibiotics in wrist arthroscopy. J Hand Surg Am 2018;43(11):987–91.e1.

42. Hulsizer D, Weiss AP, Akelman E. Ulna-shortening osteotomy after failed arthroscopic debridement of the triangular fibrocartilage complex. J Hand Surg Am 1997;22(4):694–8.

43. Sivasundaram L, Wang JH, Kim CY, et al. Emergency department utilization after outpatient hand surgery. J Am Acad Orthop Surg 2020;28(15): 639–49.

44. Verhellen R, Bain GI. Arthroscopic capsular release for contracture of the wrist: a new technique. Arthroscopy 2000;16(1):106–10.

45. Tindall A, Patel M, Frost A, et al. The anatomy of the dorsal cutaneous branch of the ulnar nerve - a safe zone for positioning of the 6R portal in wrist arthroscopy. J Hand Surg Br 2006;31(2):203–5.

46. Regal S, Tang P. Surgical management of neuromas of the hand and wrist. J Am Acad Orthop Surg 2019; 27(10):356–63.

47. Sood MK, Elliot D. Treatment of painful neuromas of the hand and wrist by relocation into the pronator quadratus muscle. J Hand Surg Br 1998;23(2): 214–9.

48. Boeckstyns ME, Sørensen AI, Viñeta JF, et al. Collagen conduit versus microsurgical neurorrhaphy: 2-year follow-up of a prospective, blinded clinical and electrophysiological multicenter randomized, controlled trial. J Hand Surg Am 2013;38(12):2405–11.

49. Guse DM, Moran SL. Outcomes of the surgical treatment of peripheral neuromas of the hand and forearm: a 25-year comparative outcome study. Ann Plast Surg 2013;71(6):654–8.

50. Adams BD, Berger RA. An anatomic reconstruction of the distal radioulnar ligaments for posttraumatic distal radioulnar joint instability. J Hand Surg Am 2002;27(2):243–51.

Triangular Fibrocartilage Complex Injuries in Children and Adolescents

Stella J. Lee, MD[a],*, Donald S. Bae, MD[b]

KEYWORDS

- Triangular fibrocartilage complex • Wrist arthroscopy • Pediatric • Ulnar-sided wrist pain

KEY POINTS

- Perform a thorough systematic examination of the wrist to evaluate for all possible causes of ulnar-sided wrist pain.
- Surgical treatment of isolated TFCC tears is considered after failure of nonoperative treatment for 3 to 6 months.
- Address all concomitant pathologies (eg, ulnocarpal impaction, distal radius malunion, or DRUJ instability) at the time of TFCC repair.
- Treatment of TFCC tears is based on the tear location (Palmer classification). The authors prefer arthroscopic-assisted outside-in repair of Palmer 1B and 1D lesions.
- Care must be taken to avoid entrapment of branches of the dorsal ulnar sensory nerve in the suture loop during TFCC repair.

INTRODUCTION

The triangular fibrocartilage complex (TFCC) serves multiple functions, transmitting axial loads across the wrist and stabilizing the distal radioulnar joint (DRUJ) during forearm rotation. As a result, the integrity of the TFCC, ulnar variance, DRUJ congruity, and DRUJ stability are interlinked. The treatment of suspected TFCC injuries in children and adolescents, and in adults, must include evaluation of all causes of ulnar-sided wrist pain.

Injuries of the TFCC have been increasingly recognized in children and adolescents in recent years. Surgical treatment continues to be guided by location of the tear as defined by the Palmer classification.[1] Multiple repair techniques, including arthroscopic-assisted methods, have been shown to result in excellent outcomes in the pediatric population with a high rate of return to sports. Additionally, proper recognition and treatment of concomitant pathologies is important to achieve the best postoperative outcomes.

ANATOMY

Descriptive Anatomy

The TFCC is a confluence of ligamentous structures that cushion the ulnocarpal articulation and stabilize the DRUJ. It is composed of the articular disk (triangular fibrocartilage proper), the meniscal homologue, dorsal and volar radioulnar ligaments, ulnolunate (UL) and ulnotriquetral (UT) ligaments, and the subsheath of the extensor carpi ulnaris (ECU) tendon (**Fig. 1**).[1–3] At its radial extent, the TFCC attaches to the distal radius distal to the sigmoid notch, then thickens dorsally and volarly to form the dorsal and volar radioulnar ligaments. Ulnarly, the deep fibers attach to the ulnar fovea and the superficial fibers attach to the ulnar carpus through its connections to the meniscal homologue.

Biomechanical Function

Biomechanically, the TFCC functions as a load-bearing and a joint-stabilizing structure. The

a Department of Surgery, Anna Jaques Hospital, 25 Highland Avenue, Newburyport, MA 01950, USA; b Boston Children's Hospital, Harvard Medical School, 300 Longwood Avenue, Fegan 2nd Floor, Boston, MA 02115, USA
* Corresponding author.
E-mail address: stella.lee@post.harvard.edu

Hand Clin 37 (2021) 517–526
https://doi.org/10.1016/j.hcl.2021.06.004

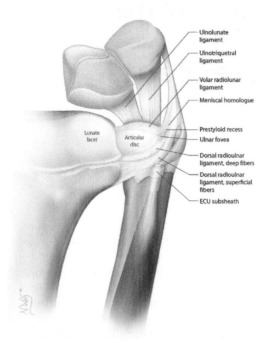

Ulnolunate ligament

Ulnotriquetral ligament

Volar radioulnar ligament

Meniscal homologue

Prestyloid recess

Ulnar fovea

Dorsal radioulnar ligament, deep fibers

Dorsal radioulnar ligament, superficial fibers

ECU subsheath

Lunate facet

Articular disc

Fig. 1. Anatomy of the triangular fibrocartilage complex. (Illustration by Nicole Wolf, MS©2020 (*nicolecwolf@gmail.com*). Printed with permission.)

hammock-like structure of the TFCC supports and stabilizes the ulnar carpus.[4] The distal ulna and TFCC bear 20% of the forces in axial loading in neutral forearm rotation in the ulnar-neutral wrist and are exposed to additional force with ulna-positive variance. Additionally, the TFCC is the major stabilizer of the DRUJ[2,5] through its attachments to the volar and dorsal radioulnar ligaments and attachment to the ulnar fovea.[6]

Cadaveric studies have demonstrated the pattern of vascularization of the TFCC, and this guides decision-making of repair versus debridement of TFCC tears. The articular disk is avascular, whereas the peripheral 15% to 20% is highly vascularized,[7] making peripheral tears amenable to surgical repair.[8]

CLINICAL PRESENTATION
Mechanism of Injury

Generally speaking, there are two mechanisms of injury: acute or primary traumatic, and degenerative or secondary to other pathology. There has been an increasing prevalence of TFCC injuries in adolescents, possibly related to increased participation in competitive sports.[9–11] The acute mechanism of injury typically involves a twisting or rotational injury, such as occurs during stick sports,[12] or from an extension-pronation force on an axially loaded hand during a fall.[9] Notably, although these injuries are typically seen in athletes, patients may not recall a specific injury[13]

preceding onset of ulnar-sided wrist pain. In a recent study, more than half of patients with a TFCC injury that underwent surgical repair had sustained a remote injury resulting in distal radius and/or ulna fracture.[14]

Clinical Presentation

Patients with TFCC tears classically complain of ulnar-sided wrist pain, which is aggravated by forceful grip, rotation of the wrist and forearm, or ulnar deviation.[15,16] Patients may also endorse mechanical symptoms of clicking and locking. However, in children and adolescents, pain may be more diffuse with a more subtle presentation[15] and may only be present during sports rather than daily activities.[9]

PHYSICAL EXAMINATION

A systematic examination of the wrist is necessary because pain can present diffusely in children. An anatomic approach to the physical examination is favored, beginning volarly and moving ulnarly, then dorsally, assessing all pathoanatomic structures: the hook of hamate, pisiform, and flexor carpi ulnaris tendon, then the ulna fovea, followed by the lunotriquetral joint, ECU tendon, and DRUJ. Examination of the contralateral side is helpful to assess for asymmetry. Starting with the unaffected side can help to gain the patient's trust. Assessment of wrist and forearm range of motion is critical and may elicit discomfort at end-range or extremes of motion.

TFCC injuries are typically associated with tenderness at the ulnar fovea, pain with end-range of supination,[12] and pain and weakness with resisted rotation. The "ulnar fovea sign" has been suggested as a key finding in patients with ulnotriquetral ligament injuries and foveal tears.[17] The TFCC compression test is a provocative test consisting of axial loading of the ulnocarpal joint with ulnar deviation and rotation.[15,18] Assessment for asymmetric clicking or clunking associated with pain is also helpful. Lunotriquetral ligament injury should be tested with lunotriquetral ballottement and shear test.[18] Because TFCC injuries and ECU tendonitis can present with pain with end-range of ulnar deviation, use of the "ECU synergy test" may help distinguish the two pathologies.[19]

Testing for DRUJ instability is critical. The DRUJ ballottement test involves passive anteroposterior and posteroanterior translation of the ulna with the radius stabilized, assessing for increased laxity and a soft end point.[6,20] However, guarding may mask instability,[6] and in the setting of an operative TFCC injury, DRUJ instability should again be assessed intraoperatively following TFCC repair.[14]

IMAGING

Plain radiographs are obtained at the time of initial evaluation to evaluate for any concomitant pathologies: malunion of prior distal radius fracture, ulnar styloid nonunion, ulnar-positive variance, or static DRUJ instability. Ulnar variance should be assessed on a zero-rotation anteroposterior view, using the "method of perpendiculars."[21]

Indications for MRI are patient-specific but may be obtained at time of initial evaluation in the setting of an acute injury with examination notable for gross instability and focal concern for TFCC injury. More typically, MRI is obtained if the patient has persistent pain after a course of nonoperative treatment.

In earlier studies, MRI had a limited role in treatment decisions, partly because of low resolution.[9] Subsequent studies have shown MR arthrography to be superior to MRI for detection of full-thickness TFCC tears, and higher field strength has been associated with higher sensitivity.[22–24] Despite increasing prevalence of 3-T MRI machines and use of surface coils,[25] more recent studies do not demonstrate increased diagnostic power of MRI. In the pediatric population, improved diagnostic power should be weighed with individual child's tolerance for injections.[18] Our current preference is for noncontrast 3-T MRI. In addition to assessing the superficial and deep fibers of the TFCC, the status of the distal radial and ulnar physes and indirect signs of symptomatic ulnocarpal impaction (eg, edema within the proximal ulnar lunate) are evaluated.

With arthroscopy findings considered the gold standard for diagnosis of TFCC tears, accuracy of MRI in diagnosing TFCC tears in children with chronic wrist pain is variable from study to study. Some studies have shown sensitivity of 94%,[26] whereas others have shown poor correlation of MRI and arthroscopic findings, with sensitivity of 29%.[27–29] It is helpful to be aware of an individual radiology department's threshold for calling abnormalities on MRI, because false-negative and false-positive rates vary across institutions.[18]

PATTERNS OF INJURY AND CLASSIFICATION

The Palmar classification, developed in 1989,[1] broadly divides TFCC injuries into traumatic (type I) and degenerative (type II) tears. Type I tears are further classified by location of TFCC tear, guiding surgical treatment. Type II tears are rare in the pediatric population. Class IA involves central perforation, class 1B avulsion from the distal ulna, class 1C volar tear with avulsion from the UL or UT ligament, and class 1D avulsion from the radial attachment at the sigmoid notch (**Box 1**). There seems to be a higher prevalence of 1B tears in children and adolescents,[9,30] with pure dorsal-ulnar or combined types comprising most TFCC tears and 1D tears the second most common tear type.[13–15] Although tear location is routinely assessed on preoperative MRI, it is confirmed with arthroscopy, and the surgeon must be prepared to address any tear type encountered intraoperatively.

More recently, there has been a growing recognition of the significance of foveal tears,[6] not included in the Palmer classification. Deep fibers of the TFCC insert into the ulnar fovea and stabilize the DRUJ. Deep fibers of the TFCC may not be clearly visualized without high-resolution MRI (**Fig. 2**), and, if left unrepaired, can lead to persistent DRUJ instability and pain. In one study, nearly half of unsatisfactory outcomes with arthroscopic TFCC repair was related to persistent DRUJ instability.[31] Integrity of the deep fibers of the TFCC should be routinely confirmed arthroscopically with a hook test. A hook is placed through the 6R or 4/5 portal into the prestyloid recess, then a radially directed traction force is applied. The test is positive if the TFCC can be displaced radially off the ulnar head.[6,28,32] Admittedly, this magnitude of injury is uncommon in the pediatric population; careful inspection of the ulnar gutter and synovial debridement is important. The

---

Box 1
Palmer classification of TFCC tears

Class 1: traumatic

A. Central perforation

B. Ulnar avulsion

C. Distal avulsion

D. Radial avulsion

Class 2: degenerative

A. TFCC wear

B. TFCC wear, lunate/ulnar chondromalacia

C. TFCC perforation, lunate/ulnar chondromalacia

D. TFCC perforation, lunate/ulnar chondromalacia, lunotriquetral (LT) ligament

E. TFCC perforation, lunate/ulnar chondromalacia, LT ligament perforation, ulnocarpal arthritis

From Palmer AK. Triangular fibrocartilage complex lesions: a classification. J Hand Surg Am. 1989;14(4):594-606. https://doi.org/10.1016/0363-5023(89)90174-3) with permission.

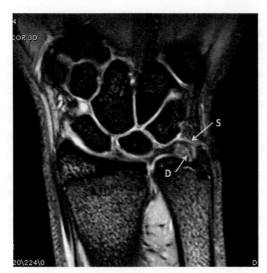

Fig. 2. High-resolution MRI may be used to detect foveal tears on imaging. In this coronal image, the superficial fibers (S) and deep fibers (D) of the TFCC are visualized. (*Courtesy of* the Children's Orthopedic Surgery Foundation, Boston MA; with permission)

importance of clinical examination and examination under anesthesia to elicit DRUJ instability cannot be overemphasized.

SURGICAL TREATMENT
Indication for Surgery

Initial treatment of TFCC tears consists of rest, activity modification, splinting, and rehabilitation with formal occupational therapy. Emphasis is placed on isometric, then isotonic, strengthening for dynamic joint stability. Indication for surgical treatment includes 4 to 6 months of nonoperative treatment with persistent pain and functional limitations with ulnar-sided pathology on MRI,[13,14] or with clinical examination and history consistent with TFCC tear. An exception is made for early surgical intervention for tears in the setting of ulnar-positive variance and ulnocarpal impaction, which typically does not improve with nonoperative treatment.

Treatment by Palmer Classification

In an early study of TFCC repairs in children and adolescents, Terry and Waters[9] recommended debridement of 1A lesions and repair of 1B, 1C, and 1D tears. The authors' current practice consists of debridement of 1A tears and repair of 1B, 1C, and 1D tears when feasible, although partial 1C and partial 1D tears may be debrided. Although there have been concerns about the vascularity of the radial aspect of the TFCC, repairs of 1D tears even in adult patients have demonstrated healing on long-term postoperative MRIs.[30] In these

situations, biologic healing and vascularity comes from the distal radius.

Other groups have advocated for debridement of radial or central tears, and combined tears resulting in large, irreparable flaps, with good results in adolescent populations.[13,33,34] Tears should be debrided to a stable rim, taking care to avoid injury to the intact foveal attachment, which can result in DRUJ instability.

Techniques of Triangular Fibrocartilage Complex Repair

Historically, TFCC tears in adolescents were repaired via an open approach.[9] More recently, several other techniques of TFCC repair ranging from all-inside knotless repairs[35] to inside-out[36] to arthroscopic-assisted outside-in repairs of 1B tears[37] and 1D tears[38] have been described in adult populations with limited comparative studies. Arthroscopic-assisted outside-in repair has shown good results in adolescents and children in several studies.[13,14,33,39] Generally speaking, arthroscopic repair is sufficient for superficial tears; in cases of DRUJ instability concerning for deep fiber foveal disruption, foveal repair or open DRUJ stabilization may yield better results. Our practice is to perform an open approach when TFCC repair is performed in conjunction with other open procedures. Open repair with transosseous suture anchor and reinforcement of the dorsal capsule has been reported in children and adolescents with good results.[40]

Concomitant Pathology

Regardless of repair technique, concomitant pathology should be addressed at the time of TFCC repair (**Fig. 3**).[9] Distal radius malunion is treated with osteotomy, and ulna-positive variance addressed with ulna-shortening osteotomy (USO).[41,42] Ulna styloid nonunion may be treated with fixation or excision. Type 2 fractures of the base of the ulna styloid lead to DRUJ instability because of loss of TFCC and ulnocarpal ligament attachments to the ulnar fovea. Treatment options include open reduction internal fixation with tension-band wiring or excision of the styloid fragment with repair of the TFCC back to the ulnar head. Restoration of DRUJ stability should be confirmed after repair.[43] Persistent DRUJ instability after TFCC repair warrants open stabilization. The Herbert sling technique,[44–46] consisting of a flap of extensor retinaculum to reconstruct the dorsal radioulnar ligament, may be used in skeletally immature patients in which a ligament reconstruction using tendon grafts and drill holes is not appropriate. Overall, there is a high rate of

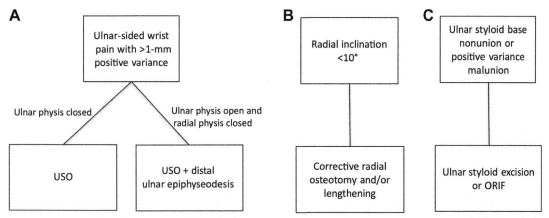

Fig. 3. Treatment algorithm for associated ulnar wrist pathologies. Surgical algorithm for performing (*A*) USO with or without distal ulnar epiphysiodesis. If the patient has clinical and/or radiographic evidence of ulnocarpal impaction and >1 mm of positive variance, USO is performed. (*B*) Corrective radial osteotomy and/or lengthening. (*C*) Ulnar styloid excision or open reduction internal fixation of ulnar styloid. ORIF, open reduction and internal fixation; USO, ulna-shortening osteotomy. (*From* Wu M. Early Results of Surgical Treatment of Triangular Fibro-cartilage Complex Tears in Children and Adolescents. J Hand Surg Am. 2020 May;45(5):449.e1-449.e9; with permission)

concomitant diagnoses warranting surgical treatment, ranging from 34% to more than 70% of TFCC repairs in some studies.[13,14,47]

Ulna-Shortening Osteotomy

USO is performed for ulna-positive variance of 1 to 2 mm or greater[14] or with evidence of ulnocarpal impaction.[13] Careful preoperative evaluation with MRI to assess for edema in the proximal ulnar aspect of the lunate may assist with decision-making (**Fig. 4**). USO may also be considered in ulna-neutral variance when 1D repairs are performed[9]; completing the osteotomy and fixation before TFCC repair improves exposure, makes 1D repair technically easier, and decreases tension on the radial side of the TFCC.[30]

Ulnar Epiphysiodesis

In patients who develop TFCC tears secondary to distal radial growth arrest and subsequent ulnar-positive variance, a distal ulnar epiphysiodesis is performed to prevent recurrent ulnar overgrowth. Through a small ulnar incision centered on the physis or extended from the prior USO incision, the distal ulnar physis is exposed with fluoroscopic confirmation. The physis may be drilled or curetted, with bone graft morselized from the segment of ulna removed at the time of shortening placed into the area, to complete the epiphysiodesis (**Fig. 5**). This additional procedure prevents recurrent deformity and avoids subsequent return of pain or TFCC injury.

Authors' Preferred Technique: 1B Tears

Type 1B repairs are completed through an outside-in approach[18,48] using a single horizontal mattress with 2–0 PDS suture (**Fig. 6**). Visualization is made through the 3/4 portal. A 4/5 portal is established to debride the ulnocarpal synovitis, which allows for visualization of the peripheral tear, and prepare the adjacent capsule. A probe is advanced into the lesion to define the extent of the tear. Using two percutaneously placed needles (TFCC Mender system, Smith and Nephew, Andover, MA), the PDS suture is passed through the capsule and through the TFCC, then back out through the TFCC in a horizontal mattress fashion, then out the capsule through the second needle. The soft tissue between the two suture limbs is carefully dissected to ensure a branch of the dorsal ulnar sensory nerve is not entrapped. To prepare for tying the suture, tension on the wrist traction tower is lessened, then the suture is tied over the joint capsule with the forearm typically in supination. Arthroscopic re-examination and palpation of the TFCC repair may be performed, but the authors do not currently routinely perform this step.

Authors' Preferred Technique: 1D Tears

We address type 1D lesions with a transradial repair[18,49] because it is a stable repair and drilling across the radius promotes vascular ingrowth into the TFCC. The lesion is probed to define the extent of the tear. The sigmoid notch is debrided in the region of the TFCC attachment. A 0.062 K-wire is

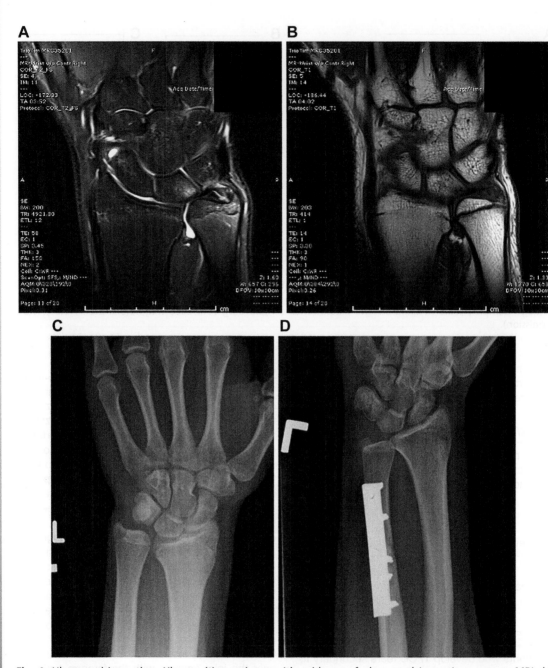

Fig. 4. Ulnocarpal impaction. Ulna-positive variance with evidence of ulnocarpal impaction seen on MRI. (*A*) There is increased signal (edema) of the distal ulna and the proximal ulnar aspect of the lunate. (*B*) Note is made of ulnar-positive variance because of a prematurely closed distal radial physis but open distal ulnar physis. (*C*) Preoperative radiograph in another patient with positive ulnar variance and TFCC tear. This patient was treated with ulna-shortening osteotomy in conjunction with TFCC repair. (*D*) Postoperative radiograph shows ulna-neutral or slightly negative variance. (*Courtesy of* the Children's Orthopaedic Surgery Foundation, Boston MA; with permission)

passed into the 6U portal, then passed through the radial edge of the TFCC and into the sigmoid notch. It is then advanced obliquely across the radius with the driver on oscillate, exiting at the radial border of the radius. A second K-wire is passed in a similar fashion, leaving a bone bridge at the radial exit point. A small longitudinal incision is made at the K-wire exit site to free up any interposed capsular tissue. Long Keith needles are used to pass a 2–0 PDS suture across the TFCC

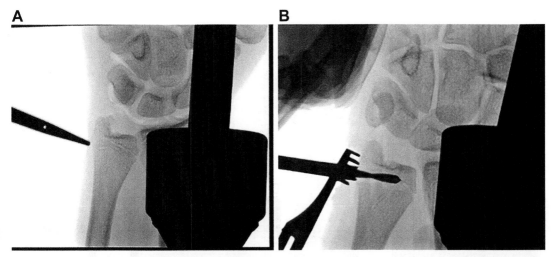

Fig. 5. Intraoperative fluoroscopy images of a distal ulnar epiphysiodesis. (*A*) The physis is confirmed via fluoroscopy. The radiopacity seen in these images is the wrist traction tower, used during wrist arthroscopy and maintained for limb positioning during the epiphysiodesis. (*B*) Drilling across the physis is performed. (*Courtesy of* the Children's Orthopaedic Surgery Foundation, Boston MA; with permission)

and across the radius, resulting in a horizontal mattress suture across the tear. Tension on the wrist traction tower is lessened, then the suture is tied over the radial bone bridge.

REHABILITATION

Postoperatively, a long arm cast is applied in supination to lessen the tension across the repair for 4 weeks, followed by a short arm cast or splint for an additional 2 weeks.[15] At 6 weeks, progressive range of motion is begun, followed by isometric strengthening, then isotonic strengthening. The patient may return to sports once full motion and full strength is achieved, typically 3 to 6 months postoperatively; in practice, children remain out of play for one entire season. Return to full sports is recommended only after sport-specific simulations in a controlled setting with minimal activity and postactivity pain.[33]

OUTCOMES

Multiple patient-report outcomes measures including Disabilities of the Arm, Shoulder and Hand (DASH), QuickDASH, modified Mayo Wrist Score, Patient-Reported Outcomes Measurement Information System (PROMIS), and Pediatric Outcomes Data Collection Instrument (PODCI) have all been used recently to track postoperative functional outcomes[13,14,33,39] with significant clinical improvement, although there may remain deficits compared with the contralateral side. Improvement in VAS pain scores is seen in most patients. In rare situations, patients may continue to have

moderate or severe pain with activity, particularly in the setting of secondary pathology (eg, chondromalacia or chondral defects).

Return to Sports

Adolescents are typically able to return to sports at 3 to 6 months postoperatively. Although most patients are typically able to return to preinjury level of play at high school or club levels,[14,33] some may return with limitations or discontinue sports entirely.[13] Expectations of return to play should be discussed with the patient and family preoperatively.

Predictors of Outcome

Improved outcomes are noted with associated bony procedures at the time of TFCC repair.[14] This has been attributed to a combination of an improved milieu for healing and treatment of all pain generators. Conversely, multiple separate operations are correlated with worse patient satisfaction, including those who undergo subsequent USO as compared with no USO or USO performed simultaneously with TFCC repair.[13]

Complications

Complications following TFCC repair include limitations in forearm rotation, need for implant removal following USO, and paresthesias in the dorsal sensory ulnar nerve distribution.[18,33,39] Dorsal sensory ulnar paresthesias are most commonly caused by traction neuropraxia, occurring in up to one out of four patients and typically resolve in 3 to

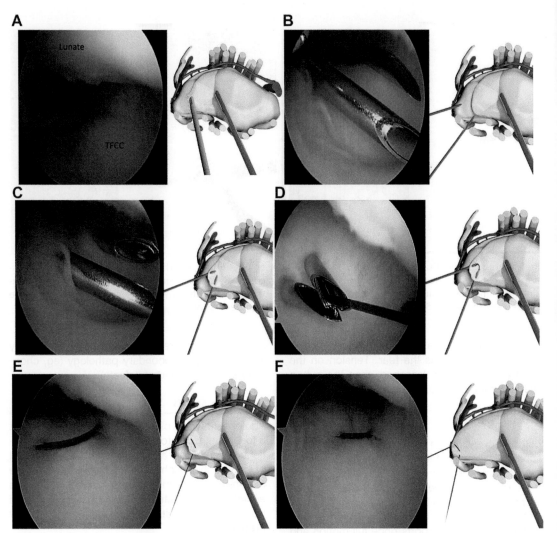

Fig. 6. Outside-in repair. Authors' preferred approach for repair of Palmer 1B lesion in a left wrist, as viewed from a 3/4 viewing portal. (*A*) The ulnar edge of the TFCC is debrided with an arthroscopic shaver. (*B*) Needles are placed percutaneously into the ulnar wrist joint. (*C*) Needles are then passed through the margin of the TFCC. (*D*) Needle bevels are turned toward each other and a 2–0 PDS suture passed. (*E*) Needles are removed, completing placement of the horizontal mattress suture. (*F*) With tension on the sutures, the TFCC is apposed to the prepared ulnar capsule. Sutures are tied down outside the capsule completing the repair, with care taken to protect branches of the dorsal ulnar sensory nerve. (*Courtesy of* the Children's Orthopaedic Surgery Foundation, Boston MA; with permission)

6 months. If there is a concern for nerve laceration or entrapment in a suture loop, this should be treated operatively without delay.[18] Notably, there is a considerable reoperation rate after TFCC repair, attributable not only to reinjuries after sports participation or symptomatic hardware but to persistent DRUJ instability or ulnocarpal impaction necessitating USO, ulnar epiphysiodesis, or distal radius osteotomy.[14,34] This underscores the need to address all pathologies at the time of the index operation.

SUMMARY

Treatment of TFCC injuries requires an understanding of its functional anatomy especially with regard to DRUJ stability. Concomitant pathologies should be addressed at the time of TFCC repair for optimal outcomes. This concept was recognized in earlier studies and has been underscored in recent studies in pediatric populations. Despite recent advances in MRI technology, variable sensitivity rates for detecting TFCC tears in children and adolescents call for surgical decision-making based heavily on clinical evaluation. Surgical treatment remains guided by the Palmer classification. There remains practice variability in the treatment methods for each tear type, but with management of concomitant wrist pathologies, repair of TFCC tears results in excellent functional outcomes in most children and adolescents.

CLINICS CARE POINTS

- Perform a thorough systematic examination of the wrist to evaluate for all possible causes of ulnar-sided wrist pain.
- Surgical treatment of isolated TFCC tears is considered after failure of nonoperative treatment for 3 to 6 months.
- Address all concomitant pathologies (eg, ulnocarpal impaction, distal radius malunion, or DRUJ instability) at the time of TFCC repair.
- Treatment of TFCC tears is based on the tear location (Palmer classification). The authors prefer arthroscopic-assisted outside-in repair of Palmer 1B and 1D lesions.
- Care must be taken to avoid entrapment of branches of the dorsal ulnar sensory nerve in the suture loop during TFCC repair.

DISCLOSURE

The authors have no conflicts of interest to disclose.

REFERENCES

1. Palmer AK. Triangular fibrocartilage complex lesions: a classification. J Hand Surg Am 1989;14(4):594–606.
2. Palmer AK, Werner FW. The triangular fibrocartilage complex of the wrist: anatomy and function. J Hand Surg Am 1981;6(2):153–62.
3. Ishii S, Palmer AK, Werner FW, et al. An anatomic study of the ligamentous structure of the triangular fibrocartilage complex. J Hand Surg Am 1998;23(6):977–85.
4. Nakamura T, Yabe Y, Horiuchi Y. Functional anatomy of the triangular fibrocartilage complex. J Hand Surg Br 1996;21(5):581–6.
5. Palmer AK, Werner FW. Biomechanics of the distal radioulnar joint. Clin Orthop Relat Res 1984;(187):26–35.
6. Atzei A, Luchetti R. Foveal TFCC tear classification and treatment. Hand Clin 2011;27(3):263–72.
7. Thiru RG, Ferlic DC, Clayton ML, et al. Arterial anatomy of the triangular fibrocartilage of the wrist and its surgical significance. J Hand Surg Am 1986;11(2):258–63.
8. Bednar MS, Arnoczky SP, Weiland AJ. The microvasculature of the triangular fibrocartilage complex: its clinical significance. J Hand Surg Am 1991;16(6):1101–5.
9. Terry CL, Waters PM. Triangular fibrocartilage injuries in pediatric and adolescent patients. J Hand Surg Am 1998;23(4):626–34.
10. Caine D, Caine C, Maffulli N. Incidence and distribution of pediatric sport-related injuries. Clin J Sport Med 2006;16(6):500–13.
11. Davis KW. Imaging pediatric sports injuries: upper extremity. Radiol Clin North Am 2010;48(6):1199–211.
12. Cornwall R. The painful wrist in the pediatric athlete. J Pediatr Orthop 2010;30:S13–6.
13. Trehan SK, Schimizzi G, Shen TS, et al. Arthroscopic treatment of triangular fibrocartilage complex injuries in paediatric and adolescent patients. J Hand Surg Eur Vol 2019;44(6):582–6.
14. Wu M, Miller PE, Waters PM, et al. Early results of surgical treatment of triangular fibrocartilage complex tears in children and adolescents. J Hand Surg Am 2020;45(5):449.e1–9.
15. Bae DS, Waters PM. Pediatric distal radius fractures and triangular fibrocartilage complex injuries. Hand Clin 2006;22(1):43–53.
16. Raskin KB, Beldner S. Clinical examination of the distal ulna and surrounding structures. Hand Clin 1998;14(2):177–90.
17. Tay SC, Tomita K, Berger RA. The "ulnar fovea sign" for defining ulnar wrist pain: an analysis of sensitivity and specificity. J Hand Surg Am 2007;32(4):438–44.
18. Bae DS, Waters PM. Pediatric hand and upper limb surgery: a practical guide. 1st edition. Philadelphia: Lippincott Williams & Wilkins; 2012. p. 657p.
19. Ruland RT, Hogan CJ. The ECU synergy test: an aid to diagnose ECU tendonitis. J Hand Surg Am 2008;33(10):1777–82.
20. Moriya T, Aoki M, Iba K, et al. Effect of triangular ligament tears on distal radioulnar joint instability and evaluation of three clinical tests: a biomechanical study. J Hand Surg Eur Vol 2009;34(2):219–23.
21. Steyers CM, Blair WF. Measuring ulnar variance: a comparison of techniques. J Hand Surg Am 1989;14(4):607–12.
22. Smith TO, Drew B, Toms AP, et al. Diagnostic accuracy of magnetic resonance imaging and magnetic resonance arthrography for triangular fibrocartilaginous complex injury: a systematic review and meta-analysis. J Bone Joint Surg Am 2012;94(9):824–32.
23. Anderson ML, Skinner JA, Felmlee JP, et al. Diagnostic comparison of 1.5 Tesla and 3.0 Tesla

preoperative MRI of the wrist in patients with ulnar-sided wrist pain. J Hand Surg Am 2008;33(7):1153–9.

24. Saupe N, Prüssmann KP, Luechinger R, et al. MR imaging of the wrist: comparison between 1.5- and 3-T MR imaging–preliminary experience. Radiology 2005;234(1):256–64.

25. Kocharian A, Adkins MC, Amrami KK, et al. Wrist: improved MR imaging with optimized transmit-receive coil design. Radiology 2002;223(3):870–6.

26. Ramavath AL, Unnikrishnan PN, George HL, et al. Wrist arthroscopy in children and adolescent with chronic wrist pain: arthroscopic findings compared with MRI. J Pediatr Orthop 2017;37(5):e321–5.

27. Gornitzky AL, Lin IC, Carrigan RB. The diagnostic utility and clinical implications of wrist MRI in the pediatric population. Hand (N Y) 2018;13(2):143–9.

28. Trehan SK, Wall LB, Calfee RP, et al. Arthroscopic diagnosis of the triangular fibrocartilage complex foveal tear: a cadaver assessment. J Hand Surg Am 2018;43(7):680.e1-5.

29. Farr S, Grill F, Ganger R, et al. Pathomorphologic findings of wrist arthroscopy in children and adolescents with chronic wrist pain. Arthroscopy 2012;28(11):1634–43.

30. Cooney WP, Linscheid RL, Dobyns JH. Triangular fibrocartilage tears. J Hand Surg Am 1994;19(1):143–54.

31. Estrella EP, Hung LK, Ho PC, et al. Arthroscopic repair of triangular fibrocartilage complex tears. Arthroscopy 2007;23(7):729–37, 737.e1.

32. Ruch DS, Yang CC, Smith BP. Results of acute arthroscopically repaired triangular fibrocartilage complex injuries associated with intra-articular distal radius fractures. Arthroscopy 2003;19(5):511–6.

33. Fishman FG, Barber J, Lourie GM, et al. Outcomes of operative treatment of triangular fibrocartilage tears in pediatric and adolescent athletes. J Pediatr Orthop 2018;38(10):e618–22.

34. Farr S, Schüller M, Ganger R, et al. Outcomes after arthroscopic debridement of the triangular fibrocartilage complex in adolescents. J Wrist Surg 2018;7(1):43–50.

35. Geissler WB. Arthroscopic knotless peripheral ulnar-sided TFCC repair. Hand Clin 2011;27(3):273–9.

36. Skie MC, Mekhail AO, Deitrich DR, et al. Operative technique for inside-out repair of the triangular

fibrocartilage complex. J Hand Surg Am 1997;22(5):814–7.

37. Whipple TL, Geissler WB. Arthroscopic management of wrist triangular fibrocartilage complex injuries in the athlete. Orthopedics 1993;16(9):1061–7.

38. Jantea CL, Baltzer A, Rüther W. Arthroscopic repair of radial-sided lesions of the triangular fibrocartilage complex. Hand Clin 1995;11(1):31–6.

39. Farr S, Zechmann U, Ganger R, et al. Clinical experience with arthroscopically-assisted repair of peripheral triangular fibrocartilage complex tears in adolescents: technique and results. Int Orthop 2015;39(8):1571e1577.

40. Pfanner S, Diaz L, Ghargozloo D, et al. TFCC lesions in children and adolescents: open treatment. J Hand Surg Asian Pac Vol 2018;23(4):506–14.

41. Trumble TE, Gilbert M, Vedder N. Ulnar shortening combined with arthroscopic repairs in the delayed management of triangular fibrocartilage complex tears. J Hand Surg Am 1997;22(5):807–13.

42. Minami A, Kato H. Ulnar shortening for triangular fibrocartilage complex tears associated with ulnar positive variance. J Hand Surg Am 1998;23(5):904–8.

43. Hauck RM, Skahen J 3rd, Palmer AK. Classification and treatment of ulnar styloid nonunion. J Hand Surg Am 1996;21(3):418–22.

44. Stanley D, Herbert TJ. The Swanson ulnar head prosthesis for post-traumatic disorders of the distal radio-ulnar joint. J Hand Surg Br 1992;17(6):682–8.

45. Dy CJ, Ouellette EA, Makowski AL. Extensor retinaculum capsulorrhaphy for ulnocarpal and distal radio-ulnar instability: the Herbert sling. Tech Hand Up Extrem Surg 2009;13(1):19e22.

46. Bauer AS, Lee SJ, Smith MD, et al. Extensor retinaculum reconstruction of the distal radioulnar joint in adolescents. Hand (N Y) 2020. https://doi.org/10.1177/1558944720966707. 1558944720966707.

47. Farr S, Grill F, Girsch W. Wrist arthroscopy in children and adolescents: a single surgeon experience of thirty-four cases. Int Orthop 2012;36(6):1215–20.

48. Frank RM, Slikker W, Al-Shihabi L, et al. Arthroscopic-assisted outside-in repair of triangular fibrocartilage complex tears. Arthrosc Techn 2015;4(5):e577ee581.

49. Sagerman SD, Short W. Arthroscopic repair of radial-sided triangular fibrocartilage complex tears. Arthroscopy 1996;12(3):339e342.

Dry Wrist Arthroscopy in the Management of Ulnar Wrist Pain Disorders

Marion Burnier, MD[a], Sanjeev Kakar, MD[b,c],*

KEYWORDS

• Ulnar wrist pain • Dry arthroscopy • TFCC • UT split Tear • Four leaf clover

KEY POINTS

- Dry wrist arthroscopy permits surgeons to expand their indications in treating disorders of the wrist.
- Ulnar wrist pain is considered to be the low back of the wrist with a myriad of different causes.
- These causes are not mutually exclusive and it is critical that the treating physician have a detailed algorithm for the diagnosis and treatment of these conditions.
- Injury of the ulnar extrinsic ligaments, such as the ulnotriquetral split tear, can be missed, which may result in recalcitrant symptoms for the patient.

INTRODUCTION

The diagnosis and treatment of ulnar-sided wrist disorders represent a challenging cause of chronic wrist pain. Given the vast array of different pathologies that can exist in such a small anatomic area, a systematic method to assess and manage these patients is needed.[1–4] Kakar and Garcia-Elias[4] devised the "Four-Leaf Clover" method to consider 4 areas that may contribute to ulnar wrist pain, as many of these causes are not mutually exclusive and treating them as such can lead to frustration for both the patient and caregiver. Another way of working up patients with ulnar wrist pain is to determine whether they have "pain only," "pain with instability," and "pain with arthritis."[3] This helps the practitioner consider the cause of the pain and what pathologies will need to be addressed concomitantly. After a thorough history and physical examination, focused imaging, including plain radiographs, computed tomography, MRI, and ultrasound scanning, may be indicated.[3,5,6] Despite these tests, arthroscopy remains the gold standard to assess and classify many causes of ulnar-sided wrist pain.[7,8]

Many use fluid insufflation to distend the joint when performing wrist arthroscopy.[9] Some of the concerns when using this technique are fluid extravasation, engorgement of the soft tissues, and distention of the joint that can cause patient pain. Dry wrist arthroscopy (DWA)[10,11] mitigates some of these factors and can be used to diagnose and treat fractures and ligament tears, and assist with fusions. Within the acute situation, such as when treating fractures, given that there is no fluid extravasation, DWA is suited to assist with fracture reduction and restoring articular congruity without the risk of compartment syndrome.[12] Given the lack of fluid extravasation, an inherent advantage of dry arthroscopy is that an open procedure can be performed concomitantly. In addition, as the joint is not being distended, larger portals can be created that facilitate the introduction of larger burrs and shavers to improve the efficiency of joint debridement.

It is important to note that there are certain occasions in which fluid insufflation is advantageous during wrist arthroscopy. This includes radiofrequency usage, as the fluid helps dissipate the heat and prevent thermal injury.[13]

a Hand and Upper Extremity Surgical Institute, Clinique du Medipole-Lyon, Villeurbanne, France;
b Department of Orthopaedic Surgery, Mayo Clinic, Rochester, MN, USA; c Department of Clinical Anatomy, Mayo Clinic, Rochester, MN, USA
* Corresponding author. Department of Orthopaedic Surgery, Mayo Clinic, Rochester, MN.
E-mail address: Kakar.Sanjeev@mayo.edu

Hand Clin 37 (2021) 527–535
https://doi.org/10.1016/j.hcl.2021.06.007

Within this article, we demonstrate the use of DWA and emphasize technical points when managing certain ulnar-sided wrist disorders. Although by no means being a complete description, we aim to highlight its diagnostic and therapeutic role in the management of triangular fibrocartilage complex (TFCC) tears, ulnar impaction syndrome, and lunotriquetral dissociation (LTD).

DRY DIAGNOSTIC ARTHROSCOPY OF THE RADIOCARPAL AND MID-CARPAL SPACES

Before starting the procedure, we routinely perform an examination under anesthesia of the uninjured and injured wrist to determine the laxity of the distal radioulnar joint (DRUJ) in neutral, pronation, and supination. This is particularly important in cases in which the functional integrity of the foveal attachment of the TFCC is in question. Sterile finger traps are then applied through the index to small fingers while the arm is suspended in a well-padded traction tower.[14,15] The tourniquet is routinely used to mitigate the risk of bleeding. Standard 3 - 4 and 6-R portals are established within the radiocarpal joint to permit a thorough arthroscopic assessment. A probe is introduced through the 6-R portal and the arthroscopic evaluation of the TFCC and adjacent structures is begun. Switching the probe and arthroscope later on allows a comprehensive assessment of the ulnar part of the radiocarpal joint.

When examining the TFCC, we perform a thorough assessment using several different maneuvers. First we look for any central or peripheral-sided tears. While using a probe, we palpate the TFCC and perform the trampoline test.[16] The test is considered positive and indicative of a tear if the natural buoyancy of the TFCC is lost. Next, the arthroscopic hook test is performed where the probe is placed under the TFCC and is pulled from ulnar to radial, thereby trying to demonstrate loss of the foveal attachment of the proximal component (deep portion) of radioulnar ligaments (RUL)[17] (**Fig. 1**). Oftentimes, the TFCC may have been torn peripherally and scarred in. Using a shaver in the 6-R portal, Greene and Kakar[18] described the "suction test" to help delineate this type of injury, which also allows the surgeon to verify successful repair of peripheral TFCC tears. It is important to use the shaver to debride any synovitis that can mask a tear especially of the volar ulnar ligaments. The volar ulnolunate and ulnotriquetral (UT) ligaments can be seen and probed from the palmar aspect of the RUL to the volar aspect of the lunate and the triquetrum, respectively, to diagnose a type 1 C TFCC injury. The pisotriquetral (PT) orifice may be seen as a small defect

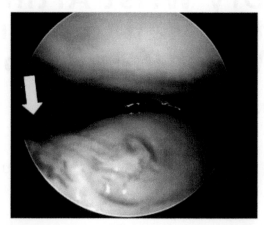

Fig. 1. Positive hook test. Note the probe (*yellow arrow*) coming from ulnar to radial lifting the TFCC from underneath, indicating foveal disruption.

in the distal aspect of the UT ligament.[19] When present, it allows a communication between the ulnocarpal and PT joints. The PT orifice is best seen by placing the arthroscope in the 6-R portal. Through this opening, the dorsal surface of the pisiform may be visualized, along with the insertion of the flexor carpi ulnaris (**Fig. 2**).

DRUJ arthroscopy can be used to assess the foveal insertion of the TFCC and the articular surfaces within the sigmoid notch.[12,20] This space can be difficult to access, and proponents of wet arthroscopy cite the use of fluid to aid in its distention between the proximal aspect of the TFCC and the distal aspect of the ulnar head.[20] Although this does hold merit, we routinely use dry arthroscopy, as we find the instilled fluid can engorge the

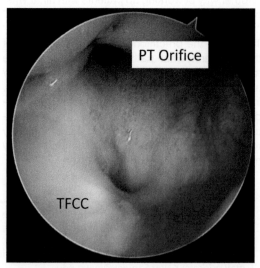

Fig. 2. Right wrist. The Pisotriquetral orifice view from the 6R portal.

synovial villi and the undersurface of the TFCC, thereby making visualization more difficult. Given that the space is limited, we do not advocate the use of a 2.7-mm arthroscope for examining the DRUJ. Instead, we use a 1.9-mm camera to examine the undersurface of the TFCC and its foveal attachments, as well as the articular surfaces within the sigmoid notch (**Fig. 3**).

When performing mid-carpal joint examination, we routinely develop the ulnar mid-carpal (MCU) portal first followed by the radial mid-carpal (MCR) portal, as sometimes, the scaphoid may be flexed secondary to a scapholunate ligament injury making the MCR space harder to access. After performing a thorough assessment of the joint, as it pertains to ulnar-sided wrist disorders, we examine for lunotriquetral (LT) instability, hamate arthrosis lunotriquetral ligament (HALT) lesions, triquetro-hamate impaction, and loose bodies/synovitis within the triquetro-hamate recess.[21]

TRIANGULAR FIBROCARTILAGE COMPLEX REPAIR

We find DWA particularly suited for the treatment of TFCC tears, as it prevents the engorgement of the soft tissues and permits DRUJ arthroscopy, as noted earlier.[22–24] Treatment depends on the arthroscopic findings and the stability of the DRUJ. Central and radial-sided tears[25] (assuming the DRUJ is stable), can be treated with debridement to a stable rim. The automatic washout technique is used to clean the joint of any debris. If radiofrequency is used, we will temporarily add fluid insufflation.

DORSAL PERIPHERAL TRIANGULAR FIBROCARTILAGE COMPLEX TEARS WITHOUT EVIDENCE OF DISTAL RADIOULNAR JOINT INSTABILITY

Oftentimes, a capsular repair can be used to treat peripheral-sided superficial TFCC tears.[9,26] Whipple and colleagues described an outside-to-inside wet arthroscopic technique to reattach dorsal peripheral tears to the floor of the sixth compartment.[9] Using a similar method, Wysocki and colleagues reported on the outcomes of 29 wrists (mean follow-up of 31 months) and noted improvements in pain and functional outcome scores, with 64% of athletes being able to return to sport.[26] One of the disadvantages of wet arthroscopy is the swelling of the soft tissues. We use a similar technique as reported and find without fluid, it makes it easier to identify and protect the dorsal sensory branch of the ulnar nerve when passing sutures.

FOVEAL TRIANGULAR FIBROCARTILAGE COMPLEX INJURY WITH DISTAL RADIOULNAR JOINT INSTABILITY

We find dry arthroscopy is particularly suited for foveal repairs. Without the instillation of fluid, we find it easier to perform DRUJ arthroscopy without engorging the synovitis or the undersurface of the TFCC. We use a modification of the technique described by Chen.[27] In brief, after performing a radiocarpal joint examination, DRUJ arthroscopy is used to confirm foveal detachment of the TFCC. An accessory working portal is then established to permit the passage of an arthroscopic shaver or curette to debride the foveal footprint. After an ulnar incision has been made, a 0.062-inch Kirschner wire (K-wire) is used to make an ulnar tunnel exiting at the fovea through which sutures are passed to capture the TFCC and permit foveal repair (**Fig. 4**).

Atzei and colleagues[28] reported an all-inside arthroscopic trans-osseous reinsertion using an anchor system. In addition to the 3 - 4, 6-R, and 6-U portals, a direct foveal (DF) portal for exploring the DRUJ is created midway between the standard proximal DRUJ and the distal DRUJ portal.[20,29] After debridement of the torn foveal

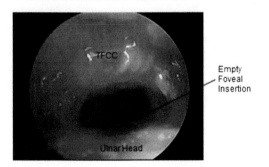

Fig. 3. Left wrist. View of an empty foveal insertion from the DRUJ portal.

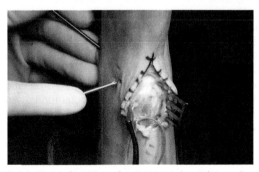

Fig. 4. Note the 6R and DRUJ portals with an ulnar incision to permit foveal debridement and arthroscopic-assisted foveal repair.

fibers to create a bleeding surface at the fovea, a suture anchor is inserted to reinsert the TFCC. In a series of 48 patients with foveal tears and DRUJ instability, the investigators reported 83.5% good to excellent Mayo Modified Wrist Scores (MMWS).[28] Pronosupination increased from 92.5% ± 13% to 99.5% ± 17%, and grip strength from 92.7% ± 19% to 103.6% ± 16% postoperatively (P<.05). DRUJ instability was persistent in 4 patients (8.3%) with a soft endpoint at the ballottement test, and 2 of them complained of the persistence of a painful click during forearm rotation. Neurapraxia of the dorsal sensory branch of the ulnar nerve occurred in 5 patients (10.4%).

Nakamura and colleagues[30] reported on an oblique trans-osseous reinsertion of the TFCC into the fovea. This outside-in trans-osseous pull-out technique can be performed freehand or with a target device inserted through the 6-R portal. Nakamura and colleagues[30] reported clinical results of 24 wrists with an average follow-up of 3.5 years. Good and excellent scores accounted for a total of 66.8%. Fifteen wrists (62.5%) reported no pain, 2 had severe pain (8.3%), and 4 had recurrent pain (16.6%).

TRIANGULAR FIBROCARTILAGE COMPLEX RECONSTRUCTION

TFCC reconstruction with tendon graft is indicated when the TFCC is considered irreparable with symptomatic DRUJ instability and without evidence of arthritis. This may happen after a neglected injury, a large tear (stage IV according to Atzei-European Wrist Arthroscopy Society [EWAS] classification[8]), or failed healing after conservative treatment or surgical repair.

Adams and Berger[31] described an open anatomic reconstruction restoring the radioulnar ligaments and their insertion into the fovea using a single graft that could be tensioned uniformly. Twelve of 14 patients had improved stability and symptoms after 1 to 4 years of follow-up.

With the advent of wrist arthroscopy, others have described their outcomes of this and similar related procedures.[32,33] Tse and colleagues[33] described a wet arthroscopic modification of the Adams and Berger[31] technique. After similar bone tunnels are created, a tendon graft is passed from dorsal to volar through the radial tunnel. An arthroscopic grasper is placed via the 4 - 5 portal between the short radiolunate and ulnolunate ligaments to retrieve the volar limb of the tendon. The graft is then passed through the ulnar bone tunnel exiting out the ulnar side. The dorsal limb is delivered into the radiocarpal joint through the 4 - 5 portal and passed into the ulnar tunnel. The graft is

then secured through a third bone tunnel made 1 cm proximal to the oblique tunnel in the ulna. Mak and Ho[34] fixed the graft using a bone tunnel in the ulna, whereas Atzei[32] preferred graft fixation with interference screw after passing the volar aspect of the tendon graft through the interval between the palmar ulnocarpal ligaments, thereby retensioning the ulnocarpal ligaments to help stabilize the ulnocarpal joint. Their outcomes are reported in **Table 1**.

ULNOTRIQUETRAL LIGAMENT SPLIT TEAR

The UT ligament is a volar structure originating from the palmar radial ulnar ligament and attaching to the palmar and ulnar triquetrum.[35,36] It can cause pain by avulsing off its attachment or developing a longitudinal split tear. Tay and colleagues[37] described the "ulnar fovea sign" as a clinical maneuver to define ulnar wrist pain by pressing dorsal and distal to the flexor carpi ulnaris tendon adjacent to the ulnar styloid. Results demonstrated a 95% sensitivity and 87% specificity for detecting foveal and/or UT ligament injuries.[37]

Oftentimes, the diagnosis of UT ligament split tears are made arthroscopically.[37,38]

Dry arthroscopy is especially useful, as the tear can be hidden underneath proliferative synovitis that can become engorged during wet arthroscopy. After arthroscopic debridement, the tear is revealed as a longitudinal split within the long axis of the UT ligament. Assuming its attachment to the triquetrum is intact, the UT ligament split tear is amenable to arthroscopic repair.[39] Tang and colleagues[40] treated 18 wrists and after a mean follow-up of 16 months, noted 63% of patients with complete resolution of pain and improvements in grip strength from 23.5 kg to 27.1 kg. Clark and colleagues[39] reported on the outcomes of 96 UT ligament split tears. After a mean follow-up of 21 months, 84% of patients achieved a good or excellent outcome in 96 UT ligament split tears. Mayo wrist scores improved from 57 to 81 after surgery, with pain scores decreasing from 5.8 to 1.2.[39] It was noted that approximately 23% of patients had additional pathology that was treated along with the UT split tear, highlighting the importance of examining for the myriad of injuries that may present in patients with ulnar wrist pain.

ULNAR IMPACTION

Symptomatic ulnar impaction can be treated via ulnar shortening (metaphyseal or diaphyseal) or wafer (open or arthroscopic) procedures. When

Table 1
Comparison of outcomes of different arthroscopic-assisted reconstruction of TFCC

	Indications	Graft Fixation	N	Mean age (Years)	Follow-up (Years)	Postop PS in Degrees (%preop)	Postop DRUJ Stable	Complications
Tse et al. 2013	Severe DRUJ Instability Irreparable TFCC	Graft around the ulna and sutured to itself	15	37	7	92° (92%)	12	3 Painful Ulnar Scar 2 Recurrences
Mak et al. 2017	Severe DRUJ Instability Irreparable TFCC	Graft around the ulna and sutured to itself	28	35	5	91° (91%)	NA	3 Painful Ulnar Scar 4 Recurrences
Luchetti-Atzei 2017	Symptomatic DRUJ Class 4 TFCC injury	Interference screw	11	37	5.5	161° (97%)	10	5 Painful Ulnar Scar 1 Recurrence 1 Ulnar Styloid Fr.

doing this arthroscopically, indications include ulnar positive variance less than 4 mm, a central TFCC tear, and no evidence of DRUJ or LT instability.[41] The arthroscope is introduced through the 3 - 4 portal while a 2.9-mm or 3.5-mm burr is placed through the 6-R portal. After debridement of the unstable TFCC flap, the top of the ulnar head from volar to dorsal is resected through the TFCC defect. We find dry arthroscopy especially useful for this procedure, as a larger skin incision can be used to permit the passage of larger, more efficient burrs. While performing the debridement, the surgeon must rotate the radius around the ulna to ensure a contoured wafer procedure is performed. We routinely use the automatic washout technique to ensure removal of the bony debris and prevent overheating of the burrs. If one is to use a radiofrequency probe to debride the TFCC, it is imperative that this is performed using saline insufflation to guard against thermal necrosis. Auzias and colleagues[42] looked at the outcomes of 33 patients treated by either diaphyseal ulnar shortening or arthroscopic wafer procedure for ulnar impaction. After a mean follow-up of 103 months in the shortening group and 55 months in the wafer group, results demonstrated similar outcomes regarding pain, grip strength, and functional outcome scores. Those patients who had an ulnar shortening osteotomy had a longer time out of work (8 months vs 4 months) and a greater number of reoperations (7 vs 3) compared with patients who had an arthroscopic wafer procedure.[42] Similar results were

reported by Oh and colleagues[41] who noted a higher complication rate in patients who had ulnar shortening procedures and improved grip strength and functional scores in the arthroscopic wafer group at 3 months after surgery. Clinical outcomes tended to be the same after 6 months of surgery.

LUNOTRIQUETRAL DISSOCIATION

LTD is a relatively common cause of ulnar-sided wrist pain. Its diagnosis and subsequent treatment can be challenging. Arthroscopy is recognized as a critical tool to evaluate the severity of lunotriquetral dissociation.[43] With the arthroscope within the MCR portal and the probe placed via an MCU portal, a step-off between the triquetrum and the lunate can be visualized. This represents an indication for stabilization after debridement if symptomatic. After assessment of cartilage damage, the evaluation of the degree of LT dissociation may be done as for the scapholunate interval using Geissler,[44,45] Dautel,[46,47] or EWAS classifications.[48,49] In an acute or subacute situation, once the debridement of the torn ligament is completed, two 0.045-inch K-wires maybe placed across the LT interval under arthroscopic and fluoroscopic control after traction is released.[50] Osterman and Seidman[50] reported on the outcomes of 20 patients without volar intercalated segment instability. After a mean of 20 months of follow-up, there was an 80% success rate with worse outcomes in those who had cartilage injury. Using a

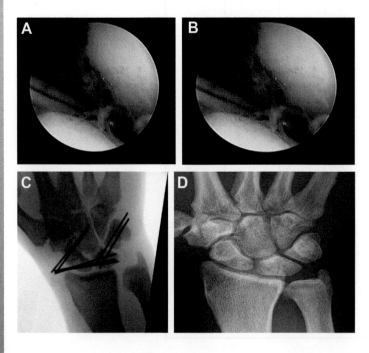

Fig. 5. Patient with a PLIND injury to the wrist. Note the gross scapholunate (A) and lunotriquetral (B) joint instability that were treated by debridement and arthroscopically guided K-wire stabilization (C). Final posteroanterior radiograph (D) showing carpus position at 10 months after surgery.

wet arthroscopic technique, Moskal and colleagues[45] described an arthroscopic stabilization of the LT joint by suture plication of the ligament and interosseous K-wire stabilization. The Mayo Wrist score increased from 50 to 88 at a mean follow-up of 3.1 years (range, 2.2–5.8 years).

For isolated LTD, combined scapholunate dissociation and perilunate instability not dislocated (PLIND) type wrist injuries (**Fig. 5**), we use DWA to assess for associated concomitant injuries including chondromalacia, and may perform concomitant dorsal capsulodesis and K-wire stabilization when indicated..[47,49]

HAMATE ARTHROSIS LUNOTRIQUETRAL INSTABILITY

Midcarpal arthritis can be associated with LT instability at the tip of the hamate.[51] This association is more often seen with type II lunates according to Viegas classification[52] and is referred to as Hamate Arthrosis Lunotriquetral Instability (HALT) syndrome. It can be treated by arthroscopic excision of the proximal pole of the hamate. Using wet techniques, Harley and colleagues[21] reported after an average of 4.7 years, 18 of 21 patients had good to excellent outcomes.

We use DWA and automatic washout techniques to perform arthroscopic resection of the proximal hamate for HALT syndrome.

SUMMARY

Apart from the use of fluid insufflation when performing thermal shrinkage procedures, we routinely use DWA to treat ulnar-sided wrist disorders. There is a minimal learning curve and it has the advantage of treating disorders without soft tissue extravasation as well as the ability to use larger, more efficient resecting instruments.

CLINICS CARE POINTS

- When treating patients with ulnar wrist pain, it is critical that the provider executes a detailed history and structured physical examination.

- Disorders of the ulnar wrist can be broken down into "bony injury," "disorders of the cartilage of the DRUJ," the status of the "dynamic stabilizers," and, finally, what is the nature of the "static stabilizers" like the TFCC.

DISCLOSURE

S. Kakar is a Consultant for Arthrex Inc but did not receive any renumeration pertaining to this article.

REFERENCES

1. Ho PC, Tse WL, Wong CW. Palmer midcarpal instability: an algorithm of diagnosis and surgical management. J Wrist Surg 2017;6(4):262–75.
2. Herzberg G. [Chronic ulnar wrist pain in adults: diagnosis and treatment principles]. Chir Main 2011;30(5):313–22.
3. Brogan DM, Berger RA, Kakar S. Ulnar-sided wrist pain: a critical analysis review. JBJS Rev 2019; 7(5):e1.
4. Kakar S, Garcia-Elias M. The "four-leaf clover" treatment algorithm: a practical approach to manage disorders of the distal radioulnar joint. J Hand Surg Am 2016;41(4):551–64.
5. Potter HG, Asnis-Ernberg L, Weiland AJ, et al. The utility of high-resolution magnetic resonance imaging in the evaluation of the triangular fibrocartilage complex of the wrist. J Bone Joint Surg Am 1997; 79(11):1675–84.
6. Victoria T, Johnson AM, Edgar JC, et al. Comparison between 1.5-T and 3-T MRI for fetal imaging: is there an advantage to imaging with a higher field strength? AJR Am J Roentgenol 2016;206(1): 195–201.
7. Palmer AK. Triangular fibrocartilage disorders: injury patterns and treatment. Arthroscopy 1990;6(2): 125–32.
8. Atzei A, Luchetti R. Foveal TFCC tear classification and treatment. Hand Clin 2011;27(3):263–72.
9. Whipple TL, Cooney WP 3rd, Osterman AL, et al. Wrist arthroscopy. Instr Course Lect 1995;44: 139–45.
10. Atzei A, Luchetti R, Sgarbossa A, et al. [Set-up, portals and normal exploration in wrist arthroscopy]. Chir Main 2006;25(Suppl 1):S131–44.
11. del Pinal F, Garcia-Bernal FJ, Pisani D, et al. Dry arthroscopy of the wrist: surgical technique. J Hand Surg Am 2007;32(1):119–23.
12. Slutsky DJ. Distal radioulnar joint arthroscopy and the volar ulnar portal. Tech Hand upper extremity Surg 2007;11(1):38–44.
13. Slutsky DJ. Wrist arthroscopy portals. Techniques in wrist and hand arthroscopy, vol 1. Elsevier; 2007. p. 1–280.
14. Herzberg G. Arthroscopie du poignet: installation, instrumentation et voies d'abord. In: Sauramps Medical, editor. L'athroscopie du Poignet. Elsevier; 2015.
15. Koo SJJ, Ho PC. Wrist arthroscopy under portal site local anesthesia without tourniquet and sedation. Hand Clin 2017;33(4):585–91.

16. Hermansdorfer JD, Kleinman WB. Management of chronic peripheral tears of the triangular fibrocartilage complex. J Hand Surg Am 1991;16(2): 340–6.

17. Ruch DS, Yang CC, Smith BP. Results of acute arthroscopically repaired triangular fibrocartilage complex injuries associated with intra-articular distal radius fractures. Arthroscopy 2003;19(5):511–6.

18. Greene RM, Kakar S. The suction test: a novel technique to identify and verify successful repair of peripheral triangular fibrocartilage complex tears. J Wrist Surg 2017;6(4):334–5.

19. Arya AP, Kulshreshtha R, Kakarala GK, et al. Visualisation of the pisotriquetral joint through standard portals for arthroscopy of the wrist: a clinical and anatomical study. J Bone Joint Surg Br 2007;89(2): 202–5.

20. Yamamoto M, Koh S, Tatebe M, et al. Arthroscopic visualisation of the distal radioulnar joint. Hand Surg 2008;13(3):133–8.

21. Harley BJ, Werner FW, Boles SD, et al. Arthroscopic resection of arthrosis of the proximal hamate: a clinical and biomechanical study. J Hand Surg Am 2004;29(4):661–7.

22. Atzei A, Rizzo A, Luchetti R, et al. Arthroscopic foveal repair of triangular fibrocartilage complex peripheral lesion with distal radioulnar joint instability. Tech Hand upper extremity Surg 2008;12(4):226–35.

23. Atzei A. New trends in arthroscopic management of type 1-B TFCC injuries with DRUJ instability. J Hand Surg Eur Vol 2009;34(5):582–91.

24. del Pinal F. The 1B constellation: an attempt to classify Palmer 1B classification. New York: Springer; 2012.

25. Bednar MS, Arnoczky SP, Weiland AJ. The microvasculature of the triangular fibrocartilage complex: its clinical significance. J Hand Surg Am 1991;16(6): 1101–5.

26. Corso SJ, Savoie FH, Geissler WB, et al. Arthroscopic repair of peripheral avulsions of the triangular fibrocartilage complex of the wrist: a multicenter study. Arthroscopy 1997;13(1):78–84.

27. Chen WJ. Arthroscopically assisted transosseous foveal repair of triangular fibrocartilage complex. Arthrosc Tech 2017;6(1):e57–64.

28. Atzei A, Luchetti R, Braidotti F. Arthroscopic foveal repair of the triangular fibrocartilage complex. J Wrist Surg 2015;4(1):22–30.

29. Atzei A. DRUJ arthroscopy. In: Operative orthopaedics of the upper extremity. New York: McGraw-Hill; 2014.

30. Nakamura T, Sato K, Okazaki M, et al. Repair of foveal detachment of the triangular fibrocartilage complex: open and arthroscopic transosseous techniques. Hand Clin 2011;27(3):281–90.

31. Adams BD, Berger RA. An anatomic reconstruction of the distal radioulnar ligaments for posttraumatic distal radioulnar joint instability. J Hand Surg Am 2002;27(2):243–51.

32. Atzei A. DRUJ instability: arthroscopic ligament reconstruction. In: del Piñal FL, Francisco, Mathoulin, editors. Arthroscopic management of ulnar pain. Springer Verlag; 2012. p. 147–60.

33. Tse WL, Lau SW, Wong WY, et al. Arthroscopic reconstruction of triangular fibrocartilage complex (TFCC) with tendon graft for chronic DRUJ instability. Injury 2013;44(3):386–90.

34. Chu-Kay Mak M, Ho PC. Arthroscopic-assisted triangular fibrocartilage complex reconstruction. Hand Clin 2017;33(4):625–37.

35. Berger RA. The anatomy of the ligaments of the wrist and distal radioulnar joints. Clin Orthop Relat Res 2001;(383):32–40.

36. Berger RA. The ligaments of the wrist. A current overview of anatomy with considerations of their potential functions. Hand Clin 1997;13(1):63–82.

37. Tay SC, Berger RA, Parker WL. Longitudinal split tears of the ulnotriquetral ligament. Hand Clin 2010;26(4):495–501.

38. Burnier M, Herzberg G, Luchetti R, et al. Dry wrist arthroscopy for ulnar-sided wrist disorders. J Hand Surg Am 2020;46(2):133–41.

39. Clark NJ, Munaretto N, Ivanov D, et al. Outcomes of ulnotriquetral split tear repair: a report of 96 patients. J Hand Surg Eur volume 2019;44(10):1036–40.

40. Tang CQY, Lai SWH, Leow G, et al. Patient-reported outcome following ulnotriquetral ligament split tear repair. J Hand Surg Asian Pac Vol 2017;22(4): 445–51.

41. Oh WT, Kang HJ, Chun YM, et al. Arthroscopic wafer procedure versus ulnar shortening osteotomy as a surgical treatment for idiopathic ulnar impaction syndrome. Arthroscopy 2018;34(2):421–30.

42. Auzias P, Delarue R, Camus EJ, et al. Ulna shortening osteotomy versus arthroscopic wafer procedure in the treatment of ulnocarpal impingement syndrome. Hand Surg Rehabil 2020;40(2):156–61.

43. Haugstvedt J. LT tears and arthroscopic repair. In: del Piñal, Francisco, Mathoulin, editors. Arthroscopic management of ulnar wrist pain. New York: Springer; 2012. p. 213–36.

44. Geissler WB, Freeland AE, Savoie FH, et al. Intracarpal soft-tissue lesions associated with an intra-articular fracture of the distal end of the radius. J Bone Joint Surg Am 1996;78(3):357–65.

45. Moskal MJ, Savoie FH 3rd, Field LD. Arthroscopic capsulodesis of the lunotriquetral joint. Clin Sports Med 2001;20(1):141–53. ix–x.

46. Dautel G, Merle M. [Dynamic arthroscopic tests for the diagnosis of scaphoid-lunar instabilities]. Ann Chir Main Memb Super 1993;12(3):206–9.

47. Herzberg G. Perilunate injuries, not dislocated (PLIND). J Wrist Surg 2013;2(4):337–45.

48. Messina JC, Van Overstraeten L, Luchetti R, et al. The EWAS classification of scapholunate tears: an anatomical arthroscopic study. J Wrist Surg 2013; 2(2):105–9.

49. Badia A, Khanchandani P. The floating lunate: arthroscopic treatment of simultaneous complete tears of the scapholunate and lunotriquetral ligaments. Hand (N Y) 2009;4(3):250–5.

50. Osterman AL, Seidman GD. The role of arthroscopy in the treatment of lunatotriquetral ligament injuries. Hand Clin 1995;11(1):41–50.

51. De Smet L. Hamate impingement: a rare cause of ulnar wrist pain ? new York: Springer; 2012.

52. Viegas SF, Wagner K, Patterson R, et al. Medial (hamate) facet of the lunate. J Hand Surg Am 1990;15(4):564–71.

LT Ligament Tears

Gregory K. Faucher, MD*, Mark Christian Moody, MD

KEYWORDS

- Lunotriquetral • Ligament • Intercarpal • Instability • Repair • Reconstruction

KEY POINTS

- Lunotriquetral (LT) ligament tears rarely occur in isolation, and diagnosis should be guided by careful history and clinical examination.
- Advanced imaging, including MR arthrogram, is useful in the diagnosis of LT tears, but arthroscopy remains the gold standard.
- Nonoperative management is appropriate for patients with partial tears and no instability.
- Repair is recommended for acute complete tears, while reconstruction is indicated for subacute and chronic cases with poor tissue quality.

INTRODUCTION

Injuries to the lunotriquetral (LT) ligament are frequently missed or misdiagnosed. These injuries are rare to occur in isolation; however, when they do, patients frequently present with normal plain radiographs. More commonly occurring radial sided carpal ligament injuries often coexist, and LT injuries occur as part of a spectrum of injuries, such as perilunate or lunate dislocations.[1] With associated injuries, the diagnosis of an LT ligament injury may be straightforward; however, in cases with isolated ulnar-sided wrist pain, LT ligament injury may not be as intuitive and should be considered.

LT ligament injuries can occur with a classic perilunate dislocation pattern, or as an isolated traumatic injury in the form of hypothenar loading in a reverse perilunate/lesser arc pattern, or can present secondary to ulnocarpal impingement in association with ulnar positive variance.[2–4] They commonly present in athletes that participate in impact sports such as football, rugby, basketball, and so forth.[5] Patients may report persistent ulnar-sided wrist pain and decreased grip strength with a history of a traumatic event. The severity of the injury can range from an LT ligament interstitial membranous tear to a complete perilunate dislocation. Treatment decisions are based on the severity of the instability and the acuity of the injury. Many patients can be treated conservatively with nonoperative management; however, surgical treatment options for acute and chronic LT ligament injuries will be discussed. Understanding the anatomy and having a heightened index of suspicion is essential to diagnose and treat these injuries successfully.

ANATOMY

The LT ligament is composed of three regions: dorsal, membranous, and volar regions.[6,7] The volar and dorsal interosseous ligaments are true ligaments with groups of parallel collagen fibers while the membranous proximal ligament is a fibrocartilaginous membrane that provides little support in terms of stability (64 N). The volar ligament is the thickest and is most important in providing resistance to palmar translation (301 N). The thinner dorsal ligament serves mainly as a restraint to rotational forces (121 N).[6,8] Dorsal translation is controlled equally by both ligaments. The LT ligament is classified as an intrinsic ligament given that its insertion is solely within the carpus. Stability of the LT ligament however relies on the surrounding bony and soft-tissue constraints that include two important extrinsic ligaments: the volar radiolunotriquetral ligament and the dorsal radiocarpal ligament.

The complex architecture of the wrist that allows for functional range of motion is beyond the scope

Division of Hand Surgery, University of South Carolina School of Medicine Greenville, Prisma Health-Upstate, The Hand Center, 1011 Frontage Drive, Greenville, SC 29615, USA
* Corresponding author.
E-mail address: Greg.Faucher@prismahealth.org

Hand Clin 37 (2021) 537–543
https://doi.org/10.1016/j.hcl.2021.06.008
0749-0712/21/© 2021 Elsevier Inc. All rights reserved.

of this article; however, it is critical to understand the linkages between the lunate, triquetrum, and their surrounding carpal bones to understand the problems that can occur as a result of LT ligament injury. The lunate has interosseus attachments to both the scaphoid through the scapholunate (SL) ligament and triquetrum through the LT ligament and, in normal anatomy, remains balanced by these opposing forces. When injury occurs to either the SL or LT ligaments, the lunate is forced to rotate with the direction of the intact ligament. The triquetrum has an articulation with the hamate that links it to the distal carpal row while the scaphoid is linked to the distal row through its articulation at the scaphotrapeziotrapezoid (STT) joint. With radial deviation, compressive forces occur at the STT joint and force the distal pole of the scaphoid to flex. The lunate along with the triquetrum follow suit through an intact SL and flex as well as translate dorsally and ulnarly. In ulnar deviation, the triquetrum's attachment with the hamate pulls the proximal row into extension through the intact LT and translates the entire proximal row radially.[9,10] This synchronous motion balances the forces seen in the midcarpal and radiocarpal joints with wrist range of motion. However, disruption of the LT or SL can lead to attritional changes in the secondary stabilizers which then leads to abnormal contact forces in the midcarpal and radiocarpal joints. As a result, volar intercalated segment instability (VISI) deformity of the proximal row can occur. Evidence of static VISI deformity implies a more global problem that involves the secondary stabilizers because sectioning of the LT alone does not result in gross radiographic evidence of the VISI position unless considerable forces are applied.[11,12] Multiple biomechanical studies endorse the importance of the volar radiolunotriquetral and dorsal radiocarpal ligament because when sectioned in association with a complete LT ligament tear, static VISI deformity is observed.[9,13,14]

Ritt and colleagues progressively destabilized the LT joint in a cadaveric study and found progressive kinematic changes.[2] They postulated that even with mildly increased mobility at the LT joint, traumatic synovitis and transfer stress can occur to surrounding tissue and articulations.[2] These findings may help to explain symptoms incurred from varying degrees of injury from partial tears to static VISI deformity and should guide treatment that will be discussed later.

PATHOPHYSIOLOGY

Multiple studies have led to a better understanding of the biomechanics of LT tears. Mayfield and colleagues[1] described the classic mechanism and classification of perilunate instability. Perilunate dislocation results from axial loading in wrist extension and ulnar deviation resulting in a progressive pattern of injury seen in **Fig. 1**. Mayfield described a lesser arc injury as being purely ligamentous and a greater arc injury pattern as involving fractures. LT tears occur at Mayfield stage III and thus would accompany multiple associated ligament or bony injuries.[1]

Another mechanism proposed by Reagan and colleagues[13] describes an injury that results in a reversed order of injury described by the Mayfield classification (**Fig. 1**B). This pattern occurs with hypothenar loading with a fall on an outstretched hand in a position of extension, protonation, and radial deviation. The ulnar-volar ligaments are then overloaded by intercarpal protonation which leads to an LT tear. The first stage of this injury pattern can result in an isolated LT tear without injury to the SL ligament.[13]

LT tears may also occur in isolation with a dorsally applied force while the wrist is in palmar flexion. The dorsal force can lead to failure of the interosseous fibers of the LT ligament while sparing the palmar radiolunotriquetral ligament.[15]

As mentioned earlier, degenerative injuries to the ulnar side of the wrist can result from ulnar positive variance due to chronic increased ulnar loading.[3,4] Ulnar abutment can cause degenerative changes, which predispose a patient to LT injury in the presence of trauma due to altered intercarpal kinematics.[3,14]

DIAGNOSIS
History and Examination

The clinical presentation of LT pathology is subtle and must be distinguished from other common sources of ulnar-sided wrist pain. Patients commonly report a fall onto outstretched hand with the wrist in extension.[13] In a study by O'Brien and colleagues,[16] 24% of patients presenting with persistent pain between one and 2 years after a fall on an outstretched hand were found to have LT instability. Point tenderness over the LT joint is a near-universal finding on examination.[13] Range of motion and grip strength should be compared to the contralateral wrist as these are commonly affected. Provocative maneuvers include the LT ballottement test and the Kleinman shear test. In the LT ballottement test, the lunate is stabilized by the thumb and index finger of one hand, while the triquetrum and pisiform are translated palmarly and then dorsally by the other. The Kleinman shear test is performed by stabilizing the dorsal aspect of the lunate with the examiner's contralateral thumb

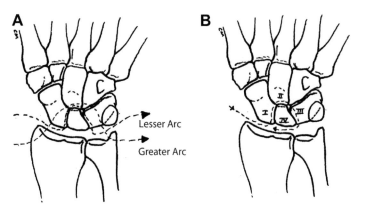

Fig. 1. (*A*) Perilunate injury. (*B*) May-field's four stages of progressive perilunate instability.

while loading the pisotriquetral joint from the palmar aspect.[17] With both maneuvers, pain, crepitus, or laxity as compared with the contralateral wrist denotes a positive test.

Imaging of the LT interval should begin with evaluation of carpal anatomy on plain radiographs. Disruption of Gilula's lines strongly suggests abnormal carpal relationships.[18] A static VISI pattern typically does not occur with isolated LT interosseous ligament disruption.[10] Dynamic VISI deformity can arise with rupture of the lunotriqetral interosseous ligament (LTIL) as well as the palmar LT ligament, while static deformity typically develops once the dorsal radiocarpal ligament has also been torn. Increased capitate-triquetrum joint distance, measured as the shortest distance between the dorsal capitate and triquetrum on neutral PA wrist radiograph can also be indicative of full-thickness LT ligament tears.[19] Clenched fist views as well as ulnar/radial deviation views can be helpful in detecting dynamic LT injuries.

Advanced imaging is useful in characterizing LT injuries, including those that are not apparent on plain radiographs. In a comparison of patients who had CT arthrography of the wrist followed by wrist arthroscopy, Bille and colleagues[20] found CT arthrography to be 85% sensitive and 79% specific when read by a radiologist and 97% sensitive and 81% specific when read by a hand surgeon. Single compartment MR arthrogram of the wrist has been shown to have a sensitivity 100% and a specificity of 94% when compared to arthroscopy.[21] 3T MRI Alone, in comparison, has been shown to have a sensitivity of 62% and a specificity of 100%.[22]

Diagnostic arthroscopy continues to be the gold standard for diagnosis of intercarpal pathology including LT ligament tears.[20–22] A useful adjunct that can be applied at the time of arthroscopy is the wrist insufflation test.[23] Before arthroscopy, the radiocarpal joint spaces are insufflated with normal saline. If there is an increased effective midcarpal joint space volume (5.6 ± 0.38 mL compromised vs 2.5 ± 0.18 mL intact) with a palpable fluid wave overlying the ulnar radiocarpal joint space, this is considered diagnostic for LT ligament tear with a sensitivity of 83.3% and specificity of 100%. Arthroscopy for evaluation of intercarpal ligament tears should include examination of both the radiocarpal and midcarpal joints. Arthroscopic grade of LT tears can be assessed using Geissler's classification system (**Table 1**).[24]

TREATMENT
Conservative Management

Conservative care should be a primary consideration in managing incomplete LT injuries and those without instability. The initial course of treatment in these cases should consist of immobilization in a forearm-based cast or splint for 6 to 8 weeks followed by progressive motion and strengthening. Nonsteroidal anti-inflammatories and ice/heat are useful adjuncts and intraarticular steroid injection can help to modulate painful synovitis. Therapy has also been investigated as a means of providing dynamic stabilization of the LT joint. The extensor carpi ulnaris (ECU) tendon acts as a midcarpal pronator, thereby inducing extension of the triquetrum.[25,26] Strengthening and proprioceptive training of the ECU, therefore, may counter the abnormal triquetral flexion seen in LT tears.

Surgical Management

Surgical intervention for LT ligament injuries is indicated when a conservative course of care fails for partial injuries or in cases of instability. A wide range of surgical options exists with limited high-level research available to help direct care. A recent systematic review showed that the majority (97%) of studies reporting outcomes for wrist ligament repair are level IV or V and that no level I or II

Table 1
Geissler arthroscopic classification of tears of the intracarpal ligaments

Grade	Description
Grade I	Attenuation or hemorrhage of interosseous ligament as seen from radiocarpal space. No incongruency of carpal alignment in mid-carpal space.
Grade II	Attenuation or hemorrhage of interosseous ligament as seen from radiocarpal space. Incongruency or step-off of carpal space. There may be a slight gap (less than width of probe) between carpal bones.
Grade III	Incongruency or step-off of carpal alignment as seen from both radiocarpal and mid-carpal space. Probe may be passed through gap between carpal bones.
Grade IV	Incongruency or step-off of carpal alignment as seen from both radiocarpal and mid-carpal space. There is gross instability with manipulation. 2.7-mm arthroscope may be passed through gap between carpal bones.

From Geissler WB, Freeland AE, Savoie FH, McIntyre LW, Whipple TL. Intracarpal Soft-Tissue Lesions Associated with an Intra-Articular Fracture of the Distal End of the Radius. *J Bone Jt Surg.* 1996;78(3):357-365. doi:10.2106/00004623-199603000-00006; with permission

studies exist.[27] Surgical intervention should be carefully tailored to each case with consideration for patient factors and injury pattern.

Arthroscopy is a mainstay of treatment and can be used both for diagnosis and management. After standard diagnostic arthroscopy, the LT interval can be approached through the ulnar-sided portals including the 4,5, 6R and midcarpal ulnar (MCU) portals. Arthroscopic debridement alone has been used as an intervention for both full and partial ligament tears. Typically, a motorized shaver is introduced through the 6R portal and used to remove unstable tissue and to create a bleeding interface between tissue and bone to facilitate healing. In one study, improved pain scores were reported in 85% of patients undergoing arthroscopic debridement only for LT, SL, and triangular fibrocartilage complex tears.[28] These results echo previously reported outcomes by Weiss and colleagues,[29] who demonstrated 100%

symptomatic improvement for patients with limited LT tears and 78% improvement for patients with complete tears after arthroscopic debridement. Electrothermal treatment of the torn ligament has also been studied as an adjunct to debridement. Pirolo and colleagues[30] demonstrated that a thermal probe can be used to effectively destroy neural tissue in the LT ligament while maintaining structural collagen, thereby denervating the injured ligament. It should be noted that these interventions do not address instability and therefore may not alleviate symptoms in patients with Geissler grade III and IV injuries.

Percutaneous pinning after debridement has been advocated for patients with instability. Once the debridement has been performed, the interval is reduced under direct visualization with an arthroscope. A probe can be used to reduce step-off at the LT interval, while K-wires can be used as joysticks to correct rotational malalignment. After reduction, two 0.045- or 0.062-in. K-wires are then passed across the interval. Pins are left for 2 months and followed with progressive mobilization with hand therapy. In a series of 20 patients with arthroscopically confirmed LT ligament tears, Ostermann and Seidman[31] reported 80% good and excellent results. In another series of 13 patients who underwent debridement and pinning for combined LT and SL injuries, 12 were pain-free and grip strength averaged 67% of contralateral at final follow-up (average 52 months).[32] This technique is primarily used in patients with Geissler grade II and III injuries.

In patients with Geissler grade IV acute LT tears, primary repair is typically recommended. Traditionally, this has been done through an open dorsal approach. The LT articulation is approached through the interval between the fourth and fifth extensor compartments, and the capsule is incised.[13] The LT interval is reduced and pinned with 0.045- or 0.062-in. K-wires. The ligament is then repaired using transosseous suture or suture anchors. The capsule can then be incorporated into the repair to restore the dorsal capsuloligamentous complex. A combined volar approach should be considered in patients with volar ligament rupture. Shin and colleagues[33] reported outcomes of primary repair with improvement of grip strength and range of motion averaging 42° of flexion and 46° of extension, but with a 13.5% probability of remaining free from complications at 5 years. More recently, all-inside arthroscopic repair of the volar capsuloligamentous complex has been described in cases in which there is enough viable tissue available for suturing.[34]

Ligament reconstruction may be a useful alternative in cases in which the residual torn ligament is not suitable for repair. These cases are typically chronic with dynamic instability. Several different techniques have been described including tenodesis, capsulodesis, and tendon grafting. Tenodesis is accomplished by passing a distally based strip of the ECU tendon through bone tunnels in the lunate and triquetrum. This has been shown to improve grip strength compared to preoperative values and to lead to superior wrist dorsiflexion when compared to repair or arthrodesis.[33] Capsulodesis for chronic LT dissociation was initially described using a 1-cm-wide radially based flap of the extensor retinaculum, sutured to the triquetrum.[35] This has been shown to yield outcomes similar to LT fusion but with lower incidence of complications and reoperation.[36] In a modification of this procedure in which the retinacular flap was fixed to both the lunate and triquetrum, good to excellent results were attained in 88% of patients when accounting for pain, patient satisfaction, grip strength, and range of motion.[37] Rather than use a retinacular flap crossing the radiocarpal joint, Omokawa and colleagues[38] sutured the dorsal radiocarpal ligament to the lunate and triquetrum using bone anchors. This was augmented with a radially based retinacular flap in cases where the dorsal radiocarpal ligament was attenuated. At average follow-up of 31 months, visual analog pain scores and Mayo wrist scores were significantly improved compared with preoperative values while range of motion and grip strength were not. Finally, palmaris longus autograft reconstruction of the deficient LT ligament has also been described.[39] In this technique, a palmaris graft is passed through "v"-patterned bone tunnels in the lunate and triquetrum, and then secured to the triquetrum and lunate using bone anchors. In a series of two patients, 83% range of motion and 91% grip strength compared to contralateral side were achieved.

LT arthrodesis is also an option for patients with chronic static instability or in those who have failed attempted soft-tissue stabilization. Multiple techniques have been described, but most include denuding the cartilage from the LT joint followed by screw, pin, or staple stabilization and bone grafting. Nonunion rates have been reported as high as 57%.[40] One study comparing tenodesis, primary repair, and arthrodesis reported decreased grip strength, wrist range of motion, and patient satisfaction in the arthrodesis group compared with tenodesis and repair.[33] Guidera and colleagues,[41] on the other hand, reported 100% union rates at an average of 50 days, with flexion/extension at 77%/80% of the contralateral side and 83% good or very good pain relief.

SUMMARY

Management of LT injures is directed by the acuity and stage of instability as well as the presence of associated injuries. Most patients without instability will do well with conservative management; however, in more severe cases, surgery may be required. Surgical planning should be tailored to each case based on patient factors, injury pattern, and degree of instability. Arthroscopy is the gold standard for diagnosis, and multiple studies have shown symptomatic improvement treating LT tears with arthroscopic debridement alone. For patients with Geissler grade II or III, we advocate arthroscopic debridement and pinning for 8 to 12 weeks. For Geissler grade IV, primary repair with or without augmentation based on available ligament for repair. For chronic instability, LT arthrodesis is an option with mixed results. Regardless of treatment, understanding the anatomy and making the correct diagnosis is essential in treating these injuries successfully.

CLINICS CARE POINTS

- Lunotriquetral (LT) ligament tears rarely occur in isolation. Static volar intercalated segment instability deformity typically develops when the dorsal radiocarpal ligament has also been torn.

- Arthroscopy remains the gold standard for diagnosis, although MR arthrogram can yield sensitivity and specificity as high as 100% and 94%, respectively.

- LT ligament injuries are graded arthroscopically using the Geissler system.

- Patients with partial tears and no instability can be treated conservatively with wrist immobilization for 6 to 8 weeks and followed by strengthening and proprioceptive training of the extensor carpi ulnaris.

- Patients with Geissler grade I and II tears may benefit from arthroscopic debridement alone. Debridement and pinning yields satisfactory results in patients with grade II and III tears.

- Primary repair should be considered for patients with Geissler grade IV complete tears. This is accomplished through an open approach using bone tunnels or suture anchors to repair the torn ligament to bone.

- In patients with chronic, static instability, ligament augmentation with capsulodesis, tenodesis, or graft has been shown to improve wrist pain and function.

- LT arthrodesis should be reserved for patients with chronic static deformities, arthrosis, or in those who have failed soft-tissue stabilization, although high rates of nonunion have been reported.

DISCLOSURE

The authors have nothing to disclose.

REFERENCES

1. Mayfield JK, Johnson RP, Kilcoyne RK. Carpal dislocations: pathomechanics and progressive perilunar instability. J Hand Surg 1980;5(3):226–41.
2. Ritt MJPF, Linscheid RL, Cooney WP, et al. The lunotriquetral joint: kinematic effects of sequential ligament sectioning, ligament repair, and arthrodesis. J Hand Surg 1998;23(3):432–45.
3. Palmer AK, Werner FW. The triangular fibrocartilage complex of the wrist—Anatomy and function. J Hand Surg 1981;6(2):153–62.
4. Mirza A, Mirza JB, Shin AY, et al. Isolated lunotriquetral ligament tears treated with ulnar shortening osteotomy. J Hand Surg 2013;38(8):1492–7.
5. Rettig AC. Athletic injuries of the wrist and hand. Am J Sports Med 2003;31(6):1038–48.
6. Ritt MJPF, Bishop AT, Berger RA, et al. Lunotriquetral ligament properties: a comparison of three anatomic subregions. J Hand Surg 1998;23(3):425–31.
7. Berger RA, Garcia-Elias M. Biomechanics of the wrist joint. In: An K, Berger RA, Cooney III WP, et al, editors. Biomechanics of the wrist joint. New York: Springer; 1991. p. 1–22.
8. Linscheid RL, Dobyns JH, Beckenbaugh RD, et al. Instability patterns of the wrist. J Hand Surg 1983; 8(5):682–6.
9. Kamal RN, Starr A, Akelman E. Carpal kinematics and kinetics. J Hand Surg 2016;41(10):1011–8.
10. Viegas SF, Patterson RM, Peterson PD, et al. Ulnar-sided perilunate instability: an anatomic and biomechanic study. J Hand Surg 1990;15(2):268–78.
11. Horii E, Garcia-Elias M, An KN, et al. A kinematic study of luno-triquetral dissociations. J Hand Surg 1991;16(2):355–62.
12. Trumble TE, Bour CJ, Smith RJ, et al. Kinematics of the ulnar carpus related to the volar intercalated segment instability pattern. J Hand Surg 1990;15(3):384–92.
13. Reagan DS, Linscheid RL, Dobyns JH. Lunotriquetral sprains. J Hand Surg 1984;9(4):502–14.
14. Sachar K. Ulnar-sided wrist pain: evaluation and treatment of triangular fibrocartilage complex tears, ulnocarpal impaction syndrome, and lunotriquetral ligament tears. J Hand Surg 2012;37(7):1489–500.
15. Alexander C, Lichtman DM. Triquetrolunate instability. In: Lichtman D, Alexander H, editors. The wrist and its disorders. 2nd edition. Philadelphia: WB Saunders; 1997. p. 307–16.
16. O'Brien L, Robinson L, Lim E, et al. Cumulative incidence of carpal instability 12-24 months after fall onto outstretched hand. J Hand Ther 2018;31(3):282–6.
17. Kleinman W. Diagnostic exams for ligamentous injuries. Chicago, Illinois: American Society for Surgery of the Hand, Correspondence Club Newsletter; 1985. p. 51.
18. Gilula L. Carpal injuries: analytic approach and case exercises. Am J Roentgenol 1979;133(3):503–17.
19. Borgese M, Boutin RD, Bayne CO, et al. Association of lunate morphology, sex, and lunotriquetral interosseous ligament injury with radiologic measurement of the capitate-triquetrum joint. Skeletal Radiol 2017;46(12):1729–37.
20. Bille B, Harley B, Cohen H. A comparison of CT arthrography of the wrist to findings during wrist arthroscopy. J Hand Surg 2007;32(6):834–41.
21. Asaad AM, Andronic A, Newby MP, et al. Diagnostic accuracy of single-compartment magnetic resonance arthrography in detecting common causes of chronic wrist pain. J Hand Surg Eur Vol 2017; 42(6):580–5.
22. Lee YH, Choi YR, Kim S, et al. Intrinsic ligament and triangular fibrocartilage complex (TFCC) tears of the wrist: comparison of isovolumetric 3D-THRIVE sequence MR arthrography and conventional MR image at 3 T. Magn Reson Imaging 2013;31(2):221–6.
23. Master DL, Yao J. The wrist insufflation test: a confirmatory test for detecting intercarpal ligament and triangular fibrocartilage complex tears. Arthrosc J Arthrosc Relat Surg 2014;30(4):451–5.
24. Geissler WB, Freeland AE, Savoie FH, et al. Intracarpal soft-tissue lesions associated with an intra-articular fracture of the distal end of the radius. J Bone Joint Surg 1996;78(3):357–65.
25. Salva-Coll G, Garcia-Elias M, Leon-Lopez MM, et al. Role of the extensor carpi ulnaris and its sheath on dynamic carpal stability. J Hand Surg Eur Vol 2011;37(6):544–8.
26. Esplugas M, Garcia-Elias M, Lluch A, et al. Role of muscles in the stabilization of ligament-deficient wrists. J Hand Ther 2016;29(2):166–74.
27. Andersson JK, Rööser B, Karlsson J. Level of evidence in wrist ligament repair and reconstruction research: a systematic review. J Exp Orthop 2018; 5(1):15.
28. Tan SW, Ng SW, Tan SH, et al. Arthroscopic debridement of intercarpal ligament and triangular fibrocartilage complex tears. Singap Med J 2012;53(3): 188–91.
29. Weiss A-PC, Sachar K, Glowacki KA. Arthroscopic debridement alone for intercarpal ligament tears. J Hand Surg 1997;22(2):344–9.

30. Pirolo JM, Le W, Yao J. Effect of electrothermal treatment on nerve tissue within the triangular fibrocartilage complex, scapholunate, and lunotriquetral interosseous ligaments. Arthrosc J Arthrosc Relat Surg 2016;32(5):773–8.

31. Osterman AL, Seidman GD. The role of arthroscopy in the treatment of lunatotriquetral ligament injuries. Hand Clin 1995;11(1):41–50.

32. Badia A, Khanchandani P. The floating lunate: arthroscopic treatment of simultaneous complete tears of the scapholunate and lunotriquetral ligaments. Hand 2009;4(3):250–5.

33. Shin AY, Weinstein LP, Berger RA, et al. Treatment of isolated injuries of the lunotriquetral ligament: a comparison of arthrodesis, ligament reconstruction and ligament repair. J Bone Joint Surg Br 2001;83-B(7):1023–8.

34. Piñal F. Arthroscopic volar capsuloligamentous repair. J Wrist Surg 2013;02(02):126–8.

35. Sennwald GR, Fischer M, Zdravkovic V. The value of arthroscopy in the evaluation of carpal instability. Bull Hosp Jt Dis 1996;54(3):186–9.

36. Smet L de, Janssens I, Ransbeeck HV. Chronic lunotriquetral dissociation: dorsal capsular reinforcement with a retinaculum flap. Acta Orthop Belg 2003;69(6):515–7.

37. Antti-Poika I, Hyrkäs J, Virkki LM, et al. Correction of chronic lunotriquetral instability using extensor retinacular split: a retrospective study of 26 patients. Acta Orthop Belg 2007;73(4):451–7.

38. Omokawa S, Fujitani R, Inada Y. Dorsal radiocarpal ligament capsulodesis for chronic dynamic lunotriquetral instability. J Hand Surg 2009;34(2):237–43.

39. Harper CM, Iorio ML. Lunotriquetral ligament reconstruction utilizing a palmaris longus autograft. J Hand Surg Asian Pac Vol 2017;22(04):544–7.

40. Sennwald GR, Fischer M, Mondi P. Lunotriquetral arthrodesis. J Hand Surg Br Eur Vol 1995;20(6):755–60.

41. Guidera PM, Watson HK, Dwyer TA, et al. Lunotriquetral arthrodesis using cancellous bone graft. J Hand Surg 2001;26(3):422–7.

Hook of Hamate Fractures

Andrea Tian, MD, Charles A. Goldfarb, MD*

KEYWORDS

• Hook of hamate • Hamate fracture • Carpal fracture • Return to play • Excision

KEY POINTS

- Hook of hamate fractures, with normal standard x-rays, may be difficult to diagnose, especially for a nonhand surgeon.
- Associated injuries may include flexor tendon rupture and ulnar nerve irritation.
- Nonoperative and operative treatment options exist. Patient and surgeon factors determine the ideal treatment option.
- Hook of the hamate excision is the widely accepted first-line treatment for most patients.
- Once correctly diagnosed and treated, hook of hamate fractures have a very good outcome with reliable return to preinjury activity levels.

INTRODUCTION

Hook of hamate fractures are relatively uncommon injuries, with reported incidence of about 2% to 4% of all carpal bone fractures.[1,2] These injuries may be difficult to diagnose, especially since most patients are often seen by nonspecialists who may initially diagnose these injuries as simple wrist sprains.[3–7] Therefore, actual incidence may be higher than reported. One population that sustains higher rates of hook of hamate fractures is athletes, specifically those that require gripping a bat/stick such as in baseball, golf, hockey, and tennis.[3,5,7–14] Stark and colleagues described the cases of 62 patients with hook of hamate fractures, 50 of whom were able to recall an event in which wrist pain occurred immediately after swinging.[3] Both operative and nonoperative treatment options exist, with hook of hamate excision being the widely accepted first line treatment for most patients. However, similar to many other orthopedic injuries, the patient's level of activity, goals of treatment, and tolerance for either surgery or immobilization must be taken into consideration.

ANATOMY

The hamate bone is the most ulnar of the distal carpal row. The hook of the hamate projects volarly from the hamate body into the palm, about 1-2 cm distal and radial to the pisiform. An easy way to palpate the hook is to place the base of one's thumb onto the pisiform and roll the thumb toward the center of the palm until the tip comes into contact with another bony prominence distally; this is the hook of the hamate (**Fig. 1**). The hook of the hamate forms the radial border of Guyon's canal and functions as the attachment site of the transverse carpal ligament, the pisohamate ligament, and the hypothenar muscles.

The ulnar nerve courses within Guyon's canal and bifurcates into superficial and deep branches. The superficial branch runs in close proximity to the tip of the hamate hook, while the deep motor branch courses along the ulnar base of the hook in direct contact with the bone.[7] Injuries to the hook of the hamate can lead to paresthesias or hypoesthesias in the ulnar nerve distribution.

Weakness in ring and small finger flexion may also be seen after hook of hamate fractures and is typically related to progressive injury to the flexor tendons as they course radially around the hook. The fracture can lead to tendon fraying and/or rupture as the tendons rub along the bony edges. Additionally, the hook has been described as a pulley for the ulnar digital flexors for increased grip strength, especially when the wrist is placed in extension and ulnar deviation.[15,16] Loss of this

Department of Orthopaedic Surgery, Washington University, 660 South Euclid Avenue, Campus Box 8233, St Louis, MO 63110, USA
* Corresponding author.
E-mail address: goldfarbc@wustl.edu

Hand Clin 37 (2021) 545–552
https://doi.org/10.1016/j.hcl.2021.06.013

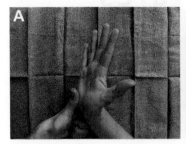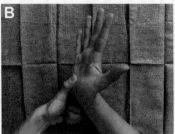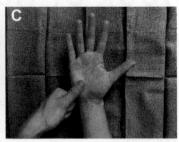

Fig. 1. Demonstration of how to palpate the hook of the hamate. (*A*) Place the base of thumb on pisiform and (*B*, *C*) roll the thumb toward center of palm until it comes into contact with another bony prominence. That is, the hook of the hamate.

fulcrum may lead to decreased excursion and, therefore, potentially decreased grip strength (**Fig. 2**).

Development

The hamate bone ossifies in the first year of life, with the hook forming from a separate, discrete ossification center.[17] The hook typically fuses to the hamate body between the ages of twelve and fifteen; failure to fuse leads to a separate ossicle termed the os hamuli proprium.[18] Unfused ossicles may be painful and can easily be confused for acute fractures, although the well-corticated, smooth edges are helpful for confirmation on radiographic imaging. The ossicles are also typically bilateral; therefore, imaging of the contralateral wrist may help distinguish a symptomatic os hamuli proprium from an acute fracture.[18,19]

Blood Supply

The blood supply to the hamate can be broken down into three regions: the dorsal nonarticular surface, the volar nonarticular surface, and the hook. In 1983, Panagis and colleagues used the modified Spateholz technique to analyze intraosseous vascularity of 25 cadaver limbs.[20] They found three to five vessels that entered the dorsal nonarticular surface and supplied the dorsal 30% to 40% of the bone. Volarly, they found one large artery that entered through the radial base of the hook that anastamosed with the dorsal vasculature. Regarding the hook, they found one to two small vessels that entered through the base and tip of the hook and anastamosed with one another, but did not anastamose with the body vasculature.[20] Similarly, Failla and colleagues used foramina found on the cortical surfaces of the hamate as a surrogate for external blood supply and found that in all 52 of their specimens, there were large foramina at the base of the hook, with 37 having foramina at the hook tip as well.[21] They posited that lack of blood flow from the tip

of the hook in 29% of their sample may contribute to development of avascular necrosis or nonunion after hook of hamate fractures.

These findings were contested by Xiao and colleagues, who stained six cadaver limbs using lead oxide and found that 27.5% of foramina did not contain blood vessels at all.[6] Their findings were similar to those of Panagis and demonstrated networks of intraosseous blood flow from both dorsal and volar nonarticular surfaces. In contrary to Panagis's findings, however, blood flow to the hook was largely from the volar nonarticular surface's network rather than a completely separate vessel. In only one of six specimens was there an artery that entered the hook from the tip. Nonetheless, all studies have agreed that the relative lack of blood flow at the midportion of the hamate hook, creating a hypovascular zone where fractures typically occur, has implications for healing potential.

HISTORY

Patients with hook of hamate fractures present with ulnar-sided wrist pain.[3,4,8–10,22] Pain is often exacerbated by grasping objects such as sporting implements, although typically does not impede other activities of daily living.[3] Reports of ulnar paresthesias are uncommon, with two of 62 patients in one cohort complaining of mild paresthesias in the small finger while four of six in another cohort had hypoesthesias of both ring and small fingers.[3,10] Flexor tendon injuries are also rare and present as weak or no flexion at the ring and/or small finger interphalangeal joints. Stark and colleagues reports an incidence of 3% (2/62) of patients who had complete ruptures of both flexor tendons to the small finger, one of whom also ruptured both tendons to the ring finger, while Bishop and Beckenbaugh cited an incidence of 19%, although this statistical includes both ruptures and fraying.[3,7] Another review of 131 cases found a tendon injury rate of 17%.[23] Interestingly, these authors report on two patients who had

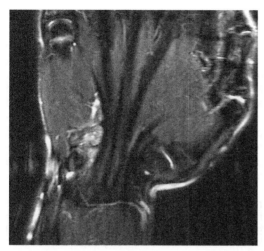

Fig. 2. MRI cut demonstrating the hook of the hamate (star) acting as a fulcrum for the flexor tendons to the ring and small fingers. Note the edema surrounding the hamate.

spontaneous tendon ruptures, one of whom could not recall any specific injury to his hand or wrist. The authors assert that spontaneous rupture of the flexor tendons to the ring or small finger should increase the clinician's suspicion of a hook of hamate fracture.

As previously mentioned, fractures of the hook of the hamate are often seen in athletes, specifically those that play baseball, hockey, golf, or tennis. When gripping the sporting tool, the base of the tool often rests against the hypothenar eminence of the supporting hand, which is often the player's nondominant hand. When the tool is used to strike a ball or puck, these forces are transferred directly onto the hook of the hamate, causing it to fracture. The classic example is the hook of the hamate fracture in the nondominant, lower batting hand in the baseball player; often there are prodromal symptoms before the acute injury/fracture.[14] These prodromal symptoms include vague, nonspecific wrist pain that comes on gradually. One tennis player noted onset of pain after changing his serving style and consequently his grip on his racquet.[24] Gradual onset of pain suggests a stress-related injury, with subsequent "acute" injury occurring through the same site. Interestingly, Yamazaki and colleagues report on three individuals who had a history of wrist injury, but whose pain had completely subsided.[25] These patients then presented to the hand surgeon's office after spontaneous flexor tendon rupture and were diagnosed with hook of hamate nonunion.[25]

Additional commonly reported mechanisms of injury involve direct blows to the palm and include

falling on an outstretched hand as well as crush injuries.[3,8,11–13,26] Some authors even report cases of patients who present to the clinic with ulnar-sided wrist pain and no recollection of prior injury.[13,23] Any patient with ulnar-sided wrist pain should be evaluated for hook of hamate fractures. A history of a direct blow to the palm or participation in batting sports should increase the clinician's suspicion.

PHYSICAL EXAM

The most commonly reported physical examination finding is tenderness over the hook of the hamate, seen in 80% to 100% of case reports.[3,7,8,12,26] Interestingly, some patients have tenderness dorsally over the hamate body as well.[7,24] Guha and Marynissen attribute this finding to the thin soft-tissue layer overlaying the dorsal hamate compared with the thick volar soft-tissue envelope superficial to the hamate hook.[24] Weakness in grip is also commonly seen and has been measured in previous reports to be about 68% to 80% that of the contralateral hand.[3,7] However, as noted previously, many athletes tend to injure their nondominant hand, as that is often the hand used to support the base of their bat/club. Therefore, grip strength may be lower at baseline.

Other physical examination findings relate to associated injuries, such as ulnar nerve irritation and flexor tendon injuries.[7,12,13,26] As with any hand injury, a good neurovascular examination is critical to understanding the patient's entire clinical picture. Special attention should be paid to the ring and small fingers when there is suspicion for hook of hamate fractures. Ulnar nerve injuries lead to paresthesias or hypoesthesias in the ulnar nerve distribution, while flexor tendon injuries lead to weakness or pain with ring/small finger flexion. Patients with complete ruptures will present with complete lack of active motion at the respective interphalangeal joints.

Because the hook of the hamate acts as a pulley around which the flexor tendons run, Wright and colleagues described the hook of hamate pull test, in which the patient flexes their ring and small fingers with the wrist held in ulnar deviation.[27] The examiner then pulls on the distal phalanxes while the patient resists extension; pain indicates a positive test.[27] The rationale behind this test is that resisted finger flexion will cause the tendons to apply an ulnarly directed force on the hook, causing fracture displacement and pain. The test was assessed on five patients whose histories were suggestive of hook of hamate fractures. All five had grossly positive results, and fractures were confirmed on computed tomography (CT) scans for all patients. This test has been used by subsequent investigators as another objective physical examination finding, although sensitivity and specificity have not yet been reported.[28]

DIAGNOSIS

Hook of hamate fractures are often initially misdiagnosed. Because these injuries are subtle, they are usually seen by a nonspecialist first and may be diagnosed as wrist sprains, triangular fibrocartilage complex injuries, or flexor carpi ulnaris tendonitis. The average time from injury to correct diagnosis in these cohorts has been reported to be from 14 weeks to 10.2 months.[3,5,7,13] In one study, the average time to diagnosis was only 27 days, although 57% of these patients were seen initially by a hand surgeon.[8]

Adding to the nonspecialist's diagnostic dilemma is the fact that hook of hamate fractures are difficult to appreciate on routine posteroanterior (PA) and lateral hand radiographs.[7,13,24,25] Only one series to our knowledge has documented success with diagnosing hook of hamate fractures using PA radiographs: Scheufler and colleagues describe a disruption of the "ring sign" that was seen in eight of 14 patients with hook of hamate fractures in their cohort.[12] A more beneficial view is the carpal tunnel view, in which the wrist is maximally dorsiflexed and the beam is aimed down the axis of the carpal tunnel. The hook forms the ulnar border of the carpal tunnel and is more easily seen in this projection (**Fig. 3**). The carpal tunnel view yields variable success, with diagnostic rates ranging from 40% to 100%.[3,7,12,25,29] However, obtaining this view may not be possible in the acute setting as a maximally dorsiflexed position can cause considerable pain to the patient.[10,24]

More recently, CT scanning has been used with increasing frequency when trying to detect hook of

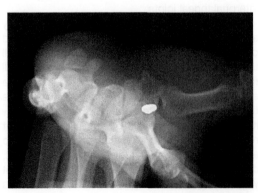

Fig. 3. Carpal tunnel view demonstrating a minimally displaced hook of hamate fracture (*arrow*).

hamate fractures. The higher definition and select cuts in three dimensions allow for 92% to 100% detection rate.[5,8,12,24,25] Magnetic resonance imaging (MRI) has shown similar success rates, although is more time-consuming and expensive. MRI can be helpful to confirm the fracture and also to assess for edema, which can be noted either before a fracture (prodromal, related to repetitive trauma) or after a fracture. The current recommendation is to perform CT scan when concerned for a possible hook of hamate fracture.[8,12,25]

Classification

Hook of hamate fractures are classified based on location. The most commonly reported location is at the base of the hook where it meets the body of the hamate, happening in 65% to 85% of fractures.[3,8,11,26] Fractures can also occur in the mid-portion or tip of the hook. Fractures at the tip of the hook are typically avulsion-type fractures.[13]

TREATMENT

Recommended treatment strategies for hook of hamate fractures vary, with both nonoperative and operative options. Choice of treatment largely depends on the patient's activity level and timeline, as well as surgeon experience. Location and timing of injury play a role as well.

Nonoperative Treatment

Owing to the fact that many hook of hamate fractures are not diagnosed accurately at the time of injury, many patients will undergo a period of nonoperative management before presenting at a hand surgeon's office. It is possible that some of these patients recover, leaving reported success rates of nonoperative management falsely low. In addition, there are reports of successful healing using casting/splinting alone. Kadar and colleagues reported on 37 patients treated nonoperatively with a success rate of 89%, although they did not list time to union and reported at least six patients who had delayed union without signs of bony bridging on CT scan at a minimum of 3 months after injury.[8] Guha and Bayer both report one case each of a nondisplaced stress fracture that healed after 6 to 8 weeks of casting.[22,24] Both athletes were able to return to their previous high level of sporting activities.

Some authors believe that the location or timing of fracture plays an important role in whether nonoperative management will be successful. Whalen and colleagues treated six acute (within

1 week of injury) fractures with casting for 6 to 12 weeks and demonstrated 100% healing at an average of 8 weeks.[26] They had similar success with one patient who was initially seen 3 weeks after onset of symptoms; this patient took 28 weeks to heal. Xiong and colleagues had greater success treating tip avulsion fractures and nondisplaced base fractures with conservative treatment and found that mid-substance fractures and displaced base fractures had better results with operative management.[13] Average time to healing with nonoperative management was about 2 months, with return to activities of daily living at 3 months and athletic activity at 5 months.[13]

The most common complication of nonoperative treatment is symptomatic nonunion. There have been multiple reports on nonunions, even in patients in whom the correct diagnosis and proper immobilization was initiated early on. These cohorts report failure rates ranging from 83% to 100%.[3,8,10,12] This is in contrast with Whalen's study, which asserted that early diagnosis and immobilization are associated with high union rates.[26] There are also reports of patients who initially appeared to heal well in a cast but had recurrence of symptoms within a few months of returning to their previous sport.[5,9] The large majority of symptomatic nonunions went on to have the fracture fragments excised with symptom resolution.[3,8,9,12]

Fracture Fragment Excision

Given the relatively poor rate of fracture union using nonoperative measures, surgical treatment is increasingly considered for patients with hook of the hamate fractures. The two widely available treatment options are fracture fragment excision and open reduction with internal fixation (ORIF). Excision involves subperiosteal dissection from a volar approach, taking care to avoid both the superficial sensory and deep motor branches of the ulnar nerve. Most authors agree that subperiosteal excision is safer than extraperiosteal for this reason.[3,5,9,12] The volar approach also allows for inspection of the flexor tendons as they course around the hamate hook (see *Flexor Tendon Injury*).

Fragment excision has shown largely favorable outcomes, with many series demonstrating 100% success rates with significant improvement in pain.[3,5,9,10,12,13,27] In these cohorts, all patients were able to return to their previous level of activities, including professional athletes, at an average of 6 to 12 weeks (see *Return to Play*). Overall patient satisfaction was rated at an average of 9.9 out of 10.[9] In contrast, Bishop and Beckenbaugh

showed only a 33% success rate, with another 33% demonstrating mild residual weakness and the final third with moderate to severe pain and weakness with gripping, altered sensation, or decreased range of motion.[7] Important to note, however, is that this study was performed in 1988, with more recent cohorts showing the previously mentioned high success rates.

Grip strength is a point of debate, with some believing that excision of the hook of the hamate reduces the excursion of the flexor tendons to the ring and small fingers, thus decreasing strength.[16] A cadaveric study showed decreased excursion by 26%, leading to a calculated 15% decrease in grip strength when the wrist is held in extension and ulnar deviation. However, this has not been shown in clinical studies.[5,12,13] In fact, Scheufler and colleagues demonstrated increased grip strength in the affected hand compared with the unaffected hand, although their cohort had the majority of injuries in the dominant hand. There have been no firm conclusions regarding absolute effect of hook excision on grip strength, yet return to play at the same level has been demonstrated in numerous studies. Overall, hook excision has good evidence of efficacy and allows patients to return to their previous level of function earlier than those who undergo treatment with casting or ORIF.[13]

Open Reduction with Internal Fixation

Another surgical treatment option for hook of hamate fractures is ORIF. Some surgeons believe that preserving the hook is important for maintaining grip strength, especially in manual laborers and athletes whose livelihoods depend on having good strength in their hands.[4,12] While ORIF can be performed from either a volar or dorsal approach, most advocate a volar approach with direct reduction and screw fixation.[12] There have been numerous reports including the use of corticocancellous bone graft, Kirschner wires, and screws.[4,7,12,13,30] Screws have gained popularity in recent years because of decreased postoperative immobilization time. Similar to hook excision, the volar approach to ORIF allows the surgeon to visualize and treat any concomitant tendon/nerve injuries. A dorsal approach has been described by Scheufler and colleagues, with cited benefits of a decreased risk of fragment devascularization, iatrogenic tendon/nerve injury, and palmar scarring.[30] ORIF has shown reasonable but not universally successful results, with union rates of 66% to 100%.[4,7,8,12,30] There are reports of persistent nonunion that required a subsequent hook excision.[7,13]

Limitations of ORIF include fracture fragment size and time to healing. The fragment must be large enough to accept a reasonably sized screw(s) for adequate fixation of the fragment.[30] Xiong and colleagues recommend ORIF only for displaced fractures at the base of the hook and avoid fixation in the mid-hook due to blood supply concerns.[13] Postoperatively, patients are immobilized for two to 3 weeks and are able to return to activities of daily living around two to 3 months, with return to sport around 5 months.[13,30] This recovery time is similar to those who undergo nonoperative management but significantly longer than the healing time for hook excision.[13]

In summary, the three major treatment options for hook of hamate fractures are immobilization in a cast/splint, fracture fragment excision, and ORIF. Immobilization alone has shown the least reliable results but remains an acceptable solution for low-demand patients who do not want or cannot undergo a surgery. ORIF has shown variable but reasonable rates of union but also requires a long period of postoperative immobilization. The procedure may be more technically challenging and requires a sufficiently large fracture fragment size as well. Hook excision is the most widely accepted treatment as it offers a straightforward surgical solution that has shown very good symptomatic relief with the shortest recovery period. It is also the salvage operation for all patients who fail nonoperative management or ORIF. While some surgeons worry that excision may lead to decreased grip strength, the current data remain equivocal and return to play rates after excision are high.

RETURN TO PLAY

As hook of hamate fractures occur predominantly in athletes, special consideration must be given to recovery time and return to play. Surgical excision is the widely accepted first-line treatment for most hook of hamate fractures given its relatively short time to recovery. Rhee and colleagues performed an analysis of Major and Minor League Baseball players and found that hook of hamate fractures were the third most common wrist injury.[31] Yet while they accounted for only 10.6% of wrist injuries, patients with hook of hamate fractures required surgery 72.4% of the time. In fact, hook of hamate excisions were the most commonly performed wrist surgery in professional baseball players. Return to play time for this cohort was found to be 51.5 days.

Other studies have found similar data. These studies included high school through professional athletes and found a mean return to play time of five to 6 weeks, regardless of level of play.[14,32] The large majority of these athletes (119/121, or 98%) were able to return to their preinjury level of performance without the need for any hand therapy. Three patients in Bansal and colleagues's cohort continued to have persistent pain despite multimodal treatment modalities.[14] With the growing pressures of year-round training and play, excision has become the treatment of choice for its restoration of preinjury performance and its quick return to play time.

COMPLICATIONS
Fracture Nonunion

As mentioned previously, one of the most common complications of hook of hamate fractures is nonunion. There are multiple theories regarding risk factors for nonunion. One theory is that many structures insert on the hook of the hamate, so as the patient moves their hand and fingers, these forces are transferred to the hook and prevent bony union.[18] In addition, the flexors of the ring and small fingers provide an ulnarly directed force to the hook. They may cause micromotion at the fracture, especially in fractures at the midsubstance of the hook.[3,13] To counteract these forces, some authors have tried using modified casts to control ring/small finger motion. Short arm casts that extend past the proximal interphalangeal joints of the ring and small fingers have not had great success achieving union.[10] However, Bayer was able to successfully treat a nondisplaced stress fracture in a cast with slight extension and radial deviation, thereby taking the ulnarly directed forces of the flexor tendons off of the fracture site.[22] In addition, there have been some studies that suggest that thumb immobilization in the form of a thumb spica cast may have greater success. This may be related to decreased thumb motion leading to decreased forces transmitted through the transverse carpal ligament onto the hook of the hamate. A cadaveric study showed that immobilization of the thumb carpometacarpal joint leads to decreased motion at the fracture site.[33] There has been one case study supporting the effectiveness of thumb spica immobilization thus far; more widespread studies are needed to analyze the true efficacy of this treatment.[34]

Flexor Tendon Injury

Flexor tendons to the ring and small finger may be injured at the time of hook of hamate fracture, or, more likely, occur secondary to fraying on a nonunited fracture. While moving tendons can displace midsubstance fractures, the fractures can also cause fraying of the tendons.[3,13,25] There are higher rates of flexor digitorum profundus ruptures than flexor digitorum superficialis.[25] At the time of surgical intervention, flexor tendons can be inspected for damage. If simply frayed, these tendons may require a debridement or no intervention at all.[9,13,27] Complete ruptures can rarely be repaired directly and often require transfers between ring and small fingers or use of palmaris/plantaris tendon grafts.[3,23,25] Injury to the flexor tendons will lead to weakness in grip strength as well as decreased range of motion, even if ruptures are repaired. Grip strength has been shown to be 86% compared with the contralateral hand, although patients are still typically satisfied with treatment and able to perform their activities of daily living.[23,25] Because of these residual deficits, some authors propose excision of fracture fragments, even if asymptomatic, to prevent the possibility of future flexor tendon ruptures.[3]

Ulnar Nerve Injury

Similar to the flexor tendons to the ring and small fingers, the superficial sensory and deep motor branches of the ulnar nerve also pass in close proximity to the hook of the hamate. To our knowledge, there has been no description of complete nerve transection secondary to hook of hamate fractures; however, there are several reports of ulnar nerve neurapraxia. Patients complain of paresthesias/hypoesthesias to the ring and/or small fingers at the time of presentation.[3,8,10,13] Electromyography can be performed preoperatively to diagnose a deep motor branch palsy, although this is not routinely performed.[7] Neurolysis is the intervention of choice for those with suspected nerve irritation and has shown good results.[13] There are some reports of transient postoperative ulnar nerve paresthesias as well as claw deformity after hook excision, all of which resolved by 5 weeks and 4 months, respectively.[5,9,14] There are no reports in the literature of permanent ulnar nerve injury after hook fracture or excision although certainly this would be the most devastating complication of surgery.

SUMMARY

Hook of hamate fractures are uncommon injuries. Presenting symptoms include ulnar-sided wrist pain, weakness in grip, or ulnar nerve paresthesias. Many of these patients are able to recall an incident in which the pain began, such as during a sporting event or after a fall onto an outstretched hand, although some have more insidious pain without a known trauma. If plain radiographs including a carpal tunnel view do not demonstrate a suspected hook of the hamate fracture, CT scan

is the recommended diagnostic tool. Hook of the hamate excision is the most widely accepted treatment option as it provides the fastest recovery time and return to play for the athlete; immobilization or ORIF can be considered for some patients. Patient factors, such as activity level and desired return to work, as well as surgeon factors, such as familiarity with surgical techniques, will shape the most appropriate treatment regimen. Once patients receive the correct diagnosis and are treated, very good outcomes with high satisfaction rates are expected.

CLINICS CARE POINTS

- Have a high suspicion for hook of hamate fractures in patients with point tenderness over the volar, ulnar hand. There may also be discomfort ulnarly or dorsally over the hamate, especially in the athlete whose pain started after striking a ball with a bat, club, and so forth.

- Perform a careful examination in all patients with suspected hook of hamate fractures, paying special attention to the flexors of the ring and small fingers as well as the deep motor branch of the ulnar nerve.

- Carpal tunnel views and computed tomography scans have the highest sensitivity for detecting hook of hamate fractures.

- Take the patient's prior activity level as well as timeline into consideration when discussing treatment options.

DISCLOSURE

The authors have nothing to disclose.

REFERENCES

1. Geissler WB. Carpal fractures in athletes. Clin Sports Med 2001;20(1):167–88.
2. van Onselen EB, et al. Prevalence and distribution of hand fractures. J Hand Surg Br 2003;28(5):491–5.
3. Stark HH, Chao EK, Zemel NP, et al. Fracture of the hook of the hamate. J Bone Joint Surg Am 1989;71(8):1202–7.
4. Watson HK, Rogers WD. Nonunion of the hook of the hamate: an argument for bone grafting the nonunion. J Hand Surg Am 1989;14(3):486–90.
5. David TS, Zemel NP, Mathews PV. Symptomatic, partial union of the hook of the hamate fracture in athletes. Am J Sports Med 2003;31(1):106–11.

6. Xiao ZR, Zhang WG, Xiong G. Features of intra-hamate vascularity and its possible relationship with avascular risk of hamate fracture. Chin Med J (Engl) 2019;132(21):2572–80.

7. Bishop AT, Beckenbaugh RD. Fracture of the hamate hook. J Hand Surg Am 1988;13(1):135–9.

8. Kadar A, Bishop AT, Suchyta MA, et al. Diagnosis and management of hook of hamate fractures. J Hand Surg Eur Vol 2018;43(5):539–45.

9. Devers BN, Douglas KC, Naik RD, et al. Outcomes of hook of hamate fracture excision in high-level amateur athletes. J Hand Surg Am 2013;38(1):72–6.

10. Egawa M, Asai T. Fracture of the hook of the hamate: report of six cases and the suitability of computerized tomography. J Hand Surg Am 1983;8(4):393–8.

11. Parker RD, Berkowitz MS, Brahms MA, et al. Hook of the hamate fractures in athletes. Am J Sports Med 1986;14(6):517–23.

12. Scheufler O, et al. Hook of hamate fractures: critical evaluation of different therapeutic procedures. Plast Reconstr Surg 2005;115(2):488–97.

13. Xiong G, Dai L, Zheng W, et al. Clinical classification and treatment strategy of hamate hook fracture. J Huazhong Univ Sci Technolog Med Sci 2010; 30(6):762–6.

14. Bansal A, Carlan D, Moley J, et al. Return to Play and Complications After Hook of the Hamate Fracture Surgery. J Hand Surg Am 2017;42(10):803–9.

15. Klausmeyer MA, Mudgal CS. Hook of hamate fractures. J Hand Surg Am 2013;38(12):2457–60 [quiz: 2460].

16. Demirkan F, Calandruccio JH, Diangelo D. Biomechanical evaluation of flexor tendon function after hamate hook excision. J Hand Surg Am 2003; 28(1):138–43.

17. Andress MR, Peckar VG. Fracture of the hook of the hamate. Br J Radiol 1970;43(506):141–3.

18. Murray WT, Meuller PR, Rosenthal DI, et al. Fracture of the hook of the hamate. AJR Am J Roentgenol 1979;133(5):899–903.

19. Wilson JN. Profiles of the Carpal Canal. J Bone Joint Surg 1954;36A(1):127–32.

20. Panagis JS, Gelberman RH, Taleisnik J, et al. The arterial anatomy of the human carpus. Part II: The intraosseous vascularity. J Hand Surg Am 1983;8(4): 375–82.

21. Failla JM. Hook of hamate vascularity: vulnerability to osteonecrosis and nonunion. J Hand Surg Am 1993;18(6):1075–9.

22. Bayer T, Schweizer A. Stress fracture of the hook of the hamate as a result of intensive climbing. J Hand Surg Eur Vol 2009;34(2):276–7.

23. Milek MA, Boulas HJ. Flexor tendon ruptures secondary to hamate hook fractures. J Hand Surg Am 1990;15(5):740–4.

24. Guha AR, Marynissen H. Stress fracture of the hook of the hamate. Br J Sports Med 2002;36(3):224–5.

25. Yamazaki H, Kato H, Nakatsuchi Y, et al. Closed rupture of the flexor tendons of the little finger secondary to non-union of fractures of the hook of the hamate. J Hand Surg Br 2006;31(3):337–41.

26. Whalen JL, Bishop AT, Linscheid RL. Nonoperative treatment of acute hamate hook fractures. J Hand Surg Am 1992;17(3):507–11.

27. Wright TW, Moser MW, Sahajpal DT. Hook of hamate pull test. J Hand Surg Am 2010;35(11):1887–9.

28. Barber JA, Loeffler B, Gaston RG, et al. Excision of Incomplete Hook of the Hamate Fractures. Orthopedics 2019;42(2):e232–5.

29. Kato H, Nakamura R, Horii E, et al. Diagnostic imaging for fracture of the hook of the hamate. Hand Surg 2000;5(1):19–24.

30. Scheufler O, Radmer S, Andresen R. Dorsal percutaneous cannulated mini-screw fixation for fractures of the hamate hook. Hand Surg 2012;17(2):287–93.

31. Rhee, CR, Camp CL, D'Angelo J, et al. Epidemiology and Impact of Hand and Wrist Injuries in Major and Minor League Baseball. Hand (N Y) 2019;16(4). 1558944719864450.

32. Burleson A, Shin S. Return to play after hook of hamate excision in baseball players. Orthop J Sports Med 2018;6(10). 2325967118803090.

33. Triplet JJ, Gellman H, Clause D, et al. The effect of thumb immobilization on fractures of the hook of the hamate: a cadaver study. Hand (N Y) 2020; 15(3):365–70.

34. Warmoth PJ, Triplet JJ, Malarkey A, et al. Thumb Immobilization in the Treatment of an Acute Hook of Hamate Fracture: A Case Report. J Long Term Eff Med Implants 2018;28(4):285–8.

Ulnocarpal Impaction

Nico Leibig, MD*, Florian M. Lampert, MD, Max Haerle, MD

KEYWORDS

- Ulnar-sided wrist pain • Ulnar shortening • Ulna abutment • Wafer procedure
- Hamate tip syndrome • Wrist arthroscopy

KEY POINTS

- Ulnocarpal impaction results from abutment between the ulnar head and the lunotriquetral complex leading to chondral changes and central or radial triangular fibrocartilage complex defects.
- Both arthroscopic wafer procedure and ulnar shortening osteotomy lead to satisfying results.
- Arthroscopic wafer procedure is more frequently indicated in elderly patients with minor ulnar plus variances (<3 mm).
- Shortening osteotomies are more frequently indicated in young patients with ulnar positive variance (>3 mm).
- Arthroscopy can be used as both a diagnostic and therapeutic tool in 1 procedure.

Video content accompanies this article at http://www.hand.theclinics.com.

BACKGROUND

In the case of a long ulna, the ulna head impacts with the carpal bones. Thereby, the triangular fibrocartilage complex (TFCC) is compressed, which leads to structural damage of the triangular articular disc in its central or radial portion. With further progression, chondral lesions of the ulnar-sided carpal bones may occur; first in the ulnar-proximal portion of the lunate and subsequently in the triquetrum. Chronic injuries may cause luno-triquetral (LT) ligament instability.

The effect of ulnar impaction syndrome (UIS) may be seen in the midcarpal joint as well, where it causes cartilage damage to the tip of the hamate, which is defined as hamate tip syndrome or hamate impingement syndrome (HIS). The assessment, pathology, and treatment options for UIS are discussed here.

Typically, UIS occurs if the ulna is long compared with the radius. Ulnar length is relatively increased by forearm pronation and grip.[1,2] With a neutral ulna, about 20% of axial load of the wrist is carried by the ulna and 80% by the radius.[3] When the ulna is 2.5 mm longer than the radius, it bears approximately 40% of axial load. UIS can still be seen in people with a neutral or even negative ulna variance.[4] These cases are usually caused by dynamic impaction of the ulna.

Most positive ulnar variance is congenital. The next most frequent cause of positive ulnar variance is secondary to shortening of the radius after a distal radius fracture.

Besides these chronic processes, acute trauma can lead to ulnocarpal impaction, when the ulnar head is compressed to the ulnar-sided carpal bones. Depending on the involved forces, this can lead to TFCC lesions as well as chondral injury.

ASSESSMENT

Usually, patients with ulnar-sided wrist pain are unable to recall a specific inciting traumatic event. On physical examination, the pain is reproduced by forearm rotation and grip testing.

Pain is typically localized just dorsal to the lunate, and a positive ulnar grinding test (pronation and supination under axial load with the wrist in

Centre for Hand and Plastic Surgery, Orthopedic Clinic Markgröningen, Kurt-Lindemann-Weg 10, 71706 Markgröningen, Germany
* Corresponding author.
E-mail address: nico.leibig@rkh-kliniken.de

Hand Clin 37 (2021) 553–562
https://doi.org/10.1016/j.hcl.2021.06.009
0749-0712/21/© 2021 Elsevier Inc. All rights reserved.

ulnar deviation) is evident. Additional tests for TFCC injuries may be positive as well, and in these cases a positive fovea sign (pressure on the soft spot between the tendons of extensor and flexor carpi ulnaris) is found. The stability of the distal radioulnar joint (DRUJ) should always be assessed.

Imaging work-up should include radiographs of the wrist in posteroanterior (PA) and lateral views. These images are performed with the shoulder abducted at 90°, the elbow flexed at 90°, and the wrist in neutral rotation. Additional functional imaging with clenched fist radiographs and with pronation are taken to reveal dynamic injuries (**Fig. 1**).

Radiographic comparison with the contralateral wrist may be helpful. Besides ulnar variance, cysts in the lunate or the ulnar head can be detected and DRUJ arthrosis or malunion of a preexisting injury should be excluded. These findings can be verified by computed tomography (CT) scans. Edema of the lunate can be seen on MRI with edema typically located at the ulnoproximal lunate, in contrast with the kienbock disease, where the disorder is located centrally or diffusely involving the entire lunate. Because of this delicate difference, ulnocarpal impaction is sometimes mistaken for kienbock disease (**Fig. 2**).

MRI may also be useful for examining TFCC lesions.[5]

DIFFERENTIAL DIAGNOSIS

Various disorders may present with similar physical examination findings to UIS, namely ulnar wrist pain. These findings include carpal arthrosis, lunotriquetral ligament injury, TFCC lesions, Essex-Lopresti injuries, kienbock disease, HIS, and DRUJ arthrosis. Sometimes, it is hard to discern one disorder from another based on physical examination, radiographs, and advanced imaging, particularly before edema or cysts are evident in the ulnar lunate. In these cases, diagnostic wrist arthroscopy is useful to delineate the disorder.

In UIS, arthroscopy reveals radial-central TFCC lesions combined with chondral changes at the lunate/hamate. In rare cases, especially in younger patients, UIS develops with an intact or often slimmed TFCC, with small chondral changes of the lunate. These patients are in an early stage of the impaction, and resection of an intact TFCC seems inappropriate.

TREATMENT
Conservative Treatment

When the ulnocarpal impaction is diagnosed, initial conservative treatment includes unloading and immobilizing the wrist combined with nonsteroidal antiinflammatory therapy.

Ulnar Shortening Osteotomy

Originally described by Milch[8] in 1941, the ulnar shortening osteotomy (USO) consists of resecting the exact amount of ulna shaft that corresponds to the ulnar positive variance. Osteosynthesis by plate fixation and postoperative immobilization is necessary to ensure bone healing. This operation has shown good results in the treatment of UIS.[6–8] The patient is typically immobilized for

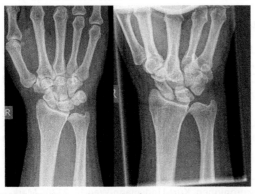

Fig. 1. (*Left*) A radiograph of a wrist in neutral position, (*right*) a clenched fist view, revealing the dynamic component of the ulnocarpal impaction. A cystic lesion is shown at the ulnar-proximal aspect of the lunate.

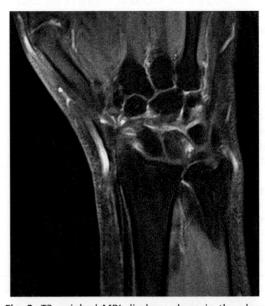

Fig. 2. T2-weighed MRI displays edema in the ulnar basis of the lunate as a consequence of the pathologic pressure of the ulnar head into the proximal carpal row.

Nonunions were the most common complications when USOs were first described with a transverse osteotomy. Some extreme cases even led to patients undergoing 1-bone forearm salvage procedures. Various studies have presented the adverse effects of smoking on osseous union after ulnar shortening.[9,10] However, nonunion rates have substantially improved secondary to advances in surgical and osteosynthesis techniques. Devices that aid by creating an oblique resection of the ulna and place a stable compression plate have greatly improved this procedure (**Fig. 4**). Even though usage of modern locking plates and screws has improved stability, reported delayed or nonunion rates are still up to 17%[10,11] (**Fig. 5**). Care must be taken in minimizing damage while resecting bone. Specifically, torsion of the distal part of the ulna is undesired because of its potential negative effect on the congruency of the DRUJ.

USO and the subsequent proximalization of the ulnar head lead to tightening of the TFCC, which additionally stabilizes the DRUJ.[12] DRUJ instability, which may be associated with ulnar positive variance, can be addressed by a USO. If instability persists, a secondary arthroscopic repair or reconstruction of the TFCC may be attempted after osseous union of the USO.[13] In these rare cases, not only TFCC injuries but also lesions of the interosseous membrane should be considered.

In order to achieve sufficient proximalization of the ulnar head during USO, the configuration of the DRUJ is critical. Tolat[14] described 3 different configurations of the DRUJ (**Fig. 6**). In Tolat C, shortening the ulna may narrow the DRUJ, leading to ulnar impingement. Preoperative evaluation of the DRUJ configuration on the PA radiograph is therefore of great importance.

In posttraumatic ulnocarpal impaction caused by shortening of the radius, the authors always consider the alternative of radial lengthening, rather than USO. In most cases, the anatomy of the distal radius determines the therapeutic

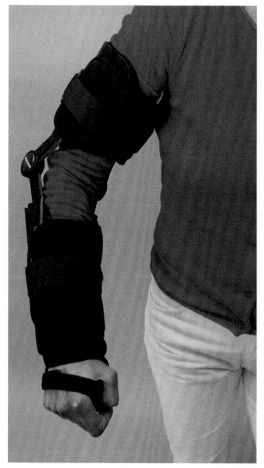

Fig. 3. Orthosis, which impedes forearm rotation while enabling elbow flexion. If required, a detachable extension for the hand splints the wrist. (*From* Sauerbier M, Eisenschenk A, Krimmer H, Partecke B-D, Schaller H-E. Die Handchirurgie. Urban & Fischer Verlag/Elsevier GmbH; 2014.; with permission)

6 weeks in a custom orthosis, which allows for elbow flexion and extension while simultaneously impeding pronation and supination (**Fig. 3**). Other investigators use a Muenster cast for this purpose.

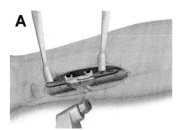 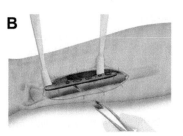 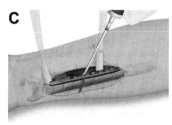

Fig. 4. (*A*) After exposure of the bone, the plate is placed onto the ulna. Using the cutting guide, a predefined slice of ulnar bone can be excised. (*B*) The plate ensures rotational stability during this procedure. (*C*) After removing the cutting guide, both fragments are compressed and the plate is locked. Using an oblique osteotomy enhances the contact surface of the bone and enables additional compression. (Courtesy of KLS Martin, Tuttlingen Germany; with permission)

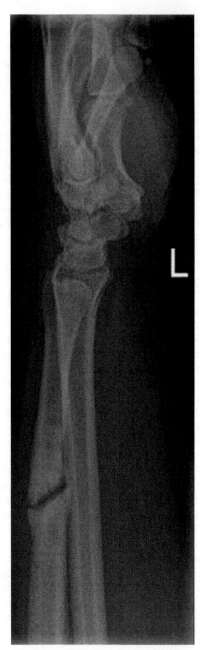

Fig. 5. Pseudarthrosis of the ulna is a feared complication of an USO. The authors recommend implant removal 2 years after osteotomy at the earliest secondary to slow bony healing.

decision. Therefore, a CT scan is recommended. If the posttraumatic shortening is combined with misalignment of the radius or incongruence of the DRUJ, a radial correction osteotomy is preferable.[15] However, if the sagittal alignment is preserved, the positive ulnar variance is treated by simple ulnar shortening (osteotomy or wafer procedure). For significant posttraumatic radius

shortening (>12 mm), a distraction osteotomy of the radius is considered[13] (**Fig. 7**).

Wafer Procedure

In 1992, Feldon and colleagues[16] described an open procedure with partial resection of a very thin slice, or wafer, of the most distal ulnar head for the treatment of UIS. The idea was to unload the ulnocarpal joint and impaction by a resection arthroplasty, without the need for postoperative immobilization and bone healing, with good results reported.[17,18] In the same year, arthroscopic wafer was introduced by Wnorowski and colleagues[19] in 9 cadaveric forearms.

During wrist arthroscopy, special attention should be paid to chondromalacia of the lunate (typically the ulnoproximal side), the triquetrum, and the ulnar head (6R portal). Stability of the luno-triquetral ligament should be tested from the ulnar midcarpal portal. Often, a central or radial irreparable TFCC lesion can be found. At least once, the diagnostic and the working portal should be switched during this procedure in order to achieve an entire overview of the wrist. Through midcarpal arthroscopy, the tip of the hamate should be examined for arthrosis.

Chondromalacia of the lunate and triquetrum, TFCC lesions, and the capsule are debrided with a shaver. Then, partial resection of the degenerative central flaps of the TFCC is recommended. This partial resection generates good access to the ulnar head. With a burr (the authors often use a 4.2 mm) the partial ulnar head resection is performed. In general, a resection of 2 to 3 mm is the maximum limit that can be achieved without negative effects to the DRUJ (**Fig. 8**).

It is essential not only to mill a notch into the ulnar head but to burr the entire semicircular ulnar head by pronating and supinating during the wafer procedure. In doing so, an oblique-helicoidal resection area is created on the ulnar head[20] (**Fig. 9**). For surgeons with limited experience, the authors recommend intraoperative radiographs in order to aid with resection (**Fig. 10**). Incomplete and oversized correction should be avoided. The DRUJ and the dorsal and palmar radioulnar ligaments can be preserved during this procedure (Video 1).

The authors prefer immobilization of the forearm for 1 week following this procedure. As in most resection arthroplasties of the wrist, satisfactory improvement is achieved after a period of 4 to 12 months postoperatively. If pain is prolonged past this period, it is likely secondary to preoperative damage to the cartilage and the load demands of the patient. The results in the literature for this

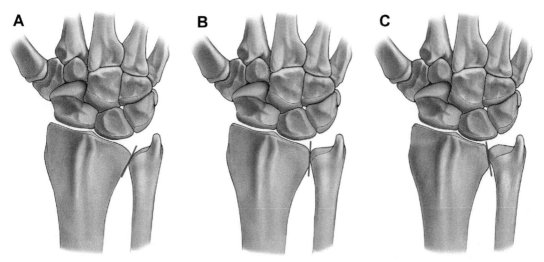

Fig. 6. The 3 different DRUJ configurations according to Tolat.[14] (*A*) In type A, the joint inclines toward the ulna. (*B*) In type B, the articular surfaces of radius and ulna run parallel. (*C*) With type C configuration, the joint inclines toward the radius. A shortening osteotomy of the ulna can narrow the joint gap in type C, leading to impingementlike symptoms. (*Modified from* Del Gaudio T, Haerle M. Die arthroskopische ulnokarpale Dekompression durch Teilresektion des Ulnakopfs. Oper Orthop Traumatol. 2016;28(4):263-269; with permission)

procedure have shown more than 80% good or excellent pain relief in more than 80% of the patients.[17,18,21]

Some investigators have discussed the pure resection of the TFCC remnants as sufficient resection arthroplasty. In rare cases, this may be a sufficient procedure, but because the TFCC is not the source of the problem, the authors still recommend resection of the ulnar head by 2 to 3 mm. An intact TFCC should not be surgically debrided in order to perform a wafer procedure.

Although preoperative MRI may show structural TFCC lesions, this does not necessarily correlate with arthroscopy. Frequently, arthroscopically proven TFCC lesions are undetected by MRI.[5,22] In these rare cases where a structurally intact

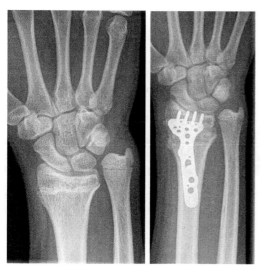

Fig. 7. Significant radial shortening (*left*), which was treated with distraction osteotomy and autologous bone grafting (*right*).

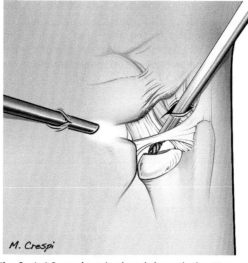

Fig. 8. A 4.2-mm burr is placed through the 6R portal for the wafer procedure. Through the 3/4 portal, the camera is introduced and, using the 30° arthroscope, an overview of the TFCC and ulnar head is seen. (*From* Sauerbier M, Eisenschenk A, Krimmer H, Partecke B-D, Schaller H-E. Die Handchirurgie. Urban & Fischer Verlag/Elsevier GmbH; 2014.; with permission)

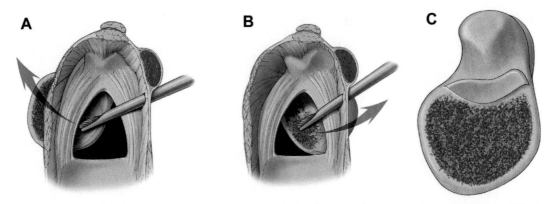

Fig. 9. During the wafer procedure, the forearm is supinated and pronated to create a homogeneous semicircular resection area with about 2 mm of depth. It is of the utmost importance during resection to preserve all articular surfaces of the DRUJ. (*From* Del Gaudio T, Haerle M. Die arthroskopische ulnokarpale Dekompression durch Teilresektion des Ulnakopfs. Oper Orthop Traumatol. 2016;28(4):263-269; with permission)

TFCC is found but signs of an impaction lesion on the proximal carpal row are seen, a USO is recommended. Only a few investigators use direct portals for arthroscopic resection of the ulnar head for these procedures. Alternatively, a mini open approach to the ulnar head resection can be performed.

Decision Making

Clinical outcomes in terms of pain relief and wrist function show comparable results for both procedures: wafer and USO.[23–25] At present, there is insufficient literature to determine indications for one or the other surgical procedure. Factors that influence this decision are the configuration of the DRUJ based on the Tolat classification, the amount of required shortening, the age of the patient, and the amount of structural damage to the TFCC.

In C-type configurations of the DRUJ, USO might create an impingement. In these cases, the wafer procedure is preferred.

Ulna positive variances greater than 3 mm tend to require an open USO. Biological healing potential of the bone is typically better in younger nonsmoking patients compared with the elderly. The wafer procedure may be more indicated for the elderly secondary to poor healing potential. If the TFCC is intact, the authors tend to preserve this entity and perform an open USO. In patients in whom radiological and clinical preoperative examination are not sufficient for ultimate decision making, a diagnostic wrist arthroscopy is indicated. While performing arthroscopy, evaluation of the points listed in **Table 1** assist us in choosing an arthroscopic wafer procedure versus open USO.

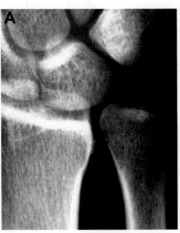

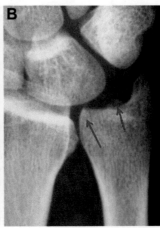

Fig. 10. Preoperatively, a pronounced positive ulna variance is shown (*A*). After a wafer procedure, the 2-mm resection (*red arrows*) is visible under radiographic visualization (*B*). Especially for less experienced providers, intraoperative radiographs are advised to avoid undercorrection or overcorrection. With increasing experience, this control can be done solely arthroscopically.

Table 1
Factors that influence the decision between open and arthroscopic shortening

	Arthroscopic Wafer Procedure	USO
TFCC	Lesion	Intact
Patient Age	Elderly	Younger
Ulnar Variance	≤3 mm	≥3 mm
DRUJ Configuration	Tolat A, B, C	Tolat A, B
Cause	Acute	Chronic

Hamate Tip Lesion

An associated injury with UIS is the hamate tip lesion. Still not completely understood, it seems to be an extension of impaction from the ulnocarpal into the midcarpal joint.[20,26,27] Alternative mechanisms for this impingement syndrome, such as midcarpal instabilities and anatomic variations (Viegas I–II), have been described.[28,29] A type II lunate according to Viegas, in which the hamate and lunate articulate, has a higher prevalence of chondromalacia of the proximal pole of the hamate.[28,30] Pain with palpation to the dorsal hamate on clinical examination and associated edema on MRI may aid in the diagnosis of this condition (**Fig. 11**).

Diagnosed is confirmed definitively by arthroscopy, which shows characteristic cartilage lesions at the tip of the hamate.[29] Treatment is performed arthroscopically by debridement of the lesion with a 3.5-mm burr (**Fig. 12**). This area is not load bearing, and resections of up to 2 mm do not alter biomechanics but relieve impingement. It was shown that resection of 2.4 mm of the proximal hamate unloads the lunate without changing the load at the triquetrohamate joint.[31]

STYLOCARPAL IMPACTION

Stylocarpal impaction, or ulnar styloid triquetral impaction, is a different form of ulnocarpal impaction. In these patients, the ulnar styloid impacts into the triquetrum, leading to pain in extension, ulnar deviation, and supination of the wrist. Wrist extension and supination cause the styloid to move closer to the triquetrum and provokes impaction. Typical movements that may trigger pain include placing the hands on the hips or back pockets or repetitively turning pages.[32] Topper and colleagues[33] described a provocation test in which the patient's hand is held in extension and pronation, followed by forearm supination while maintaining wrist extension, which may induce pain.

On clinical evaluation, tenderness is typically located at the ulnar styloid tip. Radiographs show a prominent ulnar styloid exceeding the normal 3 to 6 mm (ranging from 0 to 15 mm) and a decreased distance between ulnar styloid and triquetrum compared with the opposite side.[34] Other signs can be so-called kissing cysts in the ulnar styloid and triquetrum. Stylocarpal impaction can often be found with neutral or negative ulnar variance. Treatment options include partial styloid

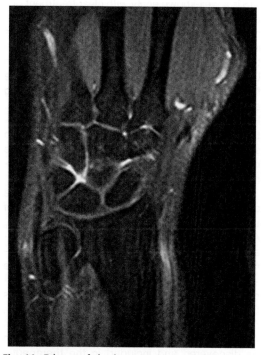

Fig. 11. Edema of the hamate tip on MRI that correlates to tenderness on the dorsal aspect of the proximal hamate on physical examination is a strong indication for HIS and should be verified arthroscopically.

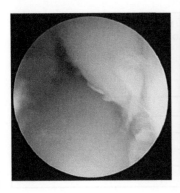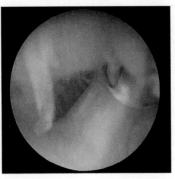

Fig. 12. In midcarpal arthroscopy, chondral lesions of the proximal hamate are detectable in HIS (*left*). Arthroscopic treatment of HIS is performed by resection of the tip of the hamate with a 3.5-mm burr (*right*).

resection by open or arthroscopic procedures. Bain and Bidwell[35] described an arthroscopy-assisted styloid resection in which a 3.5-mm burr is inserted in the 6U portal and the styloid is ablated percutaneously. Open procedures can be performed with minimal incisions. Care should be taken in reattaching the insertions of the TFCC in these procedures. However, in most cases, stylocarpal impaction is accompanied by other diagnoses, which often require other treatment.[36]

DISCUSSION

UIS is a well-known entity with clear treatment options and cause, especially with shortening secondary to a distal radius fracture.[37] The improvements of osteosynthesis and operative techniques have shown excellent results with USOs. This procedure is the operation of choice for posttraumatic patients with radial shortening and positive ulnar variance greater than 3 mm. However, USOs may lead to various complications. Specifically, the risk of ulnar nonunion should be emphasized.[17] This risk may increase if trauma, age, or nicotine abuse have compromised vascularity and bone healing potential.

Because many different disorders can cause ulnar wrist pain, the diagnosis remains one of the most challenging aspects of this condition. Arthroscopy can deliver an inside view of intra-articular lesions and is gold standard for diagnosis compared with advanced imaging. The structural damage to the cartilage, TFCC, lunotriquetral ligament, and hamate tip, as well as DRUJ instability, can be evaluated and concurrent disorders can be confirmed or excluded. Associated lesions, even if clinically silent, can be discovered and included in the therapeutic plan. In cases where the TFCC is still well attached to the fovea, USO may tighten and improve stabilization of the DRUJ while simultaneously shortening the ulna.

There are several advantages of the arthroscopic wafer procedure, compared with the open USO. It provides the benefits of being minimally invasive, with less morbidity, earlier motion, less recovery time, earlier return to work, and greater patient acceptance.[29] Because of these benefits, this operation is especially suitable for elderly patients and does not involve the risk of nonunion, as with a USO. In contrast, note that, in all long-standing chronic impaction syndromes, complete relief of any symptoms made take up to 1 year after elimination of the impaction causes. Another advantage of arthroscopy is the opportunity to address associated lesions or structural changes in the same operation. The degenerated elements, and especially the TFCC, can be debrided. Alternative forms of impaction syndrome such as styloid impaction or hamate tip syndrome can be addressed during the same arthroscopic procedure. Studies have shown that, after arthroscopic procedures, complications and revision surgeries were less often required.[21] However, a possible complication of the wafer procedure is incomplete or insufficient resection. One drawback of the wafer procedure is that ulnar shortening is only possible up to 2 to 3 mm.

Contrarily, the treatment of hamate tip syndrome, which may also be addressed arthroscopically, is not as well developed. Even if minimal arthroscopic resections have given excellent results, long-term studies need to be performed to determine the exact clinical sequelae of excision of the proximal pole of the hamate, specifically on the biomechanics of the triquetrohamate articulation.[29]

SUMMARY

Ulna plus variances greater than 3 mm should be treated by USO. Ulna plus variances associated with malunion of the distal radius should be treated by corrective osteotomy of the distal radius. Diagnosis can generally be made by radiographs and

MRI. Arthroscopy can confirm diagnosis and detect or exclude associated lesions. An arthroscopic wafer procedure gives good results in ulna plus variances less than 3 mm. Associated lesions or other disorders leading to impaction can be addressed during the same arthroscopic surgery.

Factors that influence decision making between arthroscopic and open surgical procedures are the amount of ulna positive variance, the age of the patient, the structural damage to the TFCC, and the configuration of the DRUJ.

CLINICS CARE POINTS

- Ulnocarpal impaction syndrome consists of pathologic abutment between the ulnar head and the lunotriquetral complex.
- This condition may lead to chondral changes of the lunate and triquetrum as well as radial TFCC lesions.
- Ulnocarpal impaction is a common cause for ulnar-sided wrist pain.
- Pain is typically triggered by load bearing and rotation of the forearm.
- Radiographic examination is often associated with positive ulnar variance and cysts in the lunate.
- MRI may show edema of the lunate and occasionally of the proximal hamate.
- Operative treatment aims to reduce load on the lunate.
- Both the arthroscopic wafer procedure and USO lead to satisfying results.
- Arthroscopic wafer procedure is more frequently indicated in elderly patients with minor ulnar positive variance (<3 mm).
- Shortening osteotomies are more frequently indicated in young patients with ulnar positive variance (>3 mm).
- Arthroscopy can be used as a diagnostic and therapeutic tool.

DISCLOSURE

Prof. Dr. M. Haerle is working as a medical adviser for Karl Storz, Germany and KLS Martin, Germany.

SUPPLEMENTARY DATA

Supplementary data to this article can be found online at https://doi.org/10.1016/j.hcl.2021.06.009.

REFERENCES

1. Tomaino MM. The importance of the pronated grip x-ray view in evaluating ulnar variance. J Hand Surg Am 2000;25(2):352–7.
2. Tomaino MM, Rubin DA. The value of the pronated-grip view radiograph in assessing dynamic ulnar positive variance: a case report. Am J Orthop 1999;28(3):180–1.
3. Palmer AK, Werner FW. Biomechanics of the distal radioulnar joint. Clin Orthop Relat Res 1984;187: 26–35.
4. Tomaino MM. Ulnar impaction syndrome in the ulnar negative and neutral wrist. Diagnosis and pathoanatomy. J Hand Surg Br 1998;23(6):754–7.
5. Schmauss D, Pöhlmann S, Lohmeyer JA, et al. Clinical tests and magnetic resonance imaging have limited diagnostic value for triangular fibrocartilaginous complex lesions. Arch Orthop Trauma Surg 2016;136(6): 873–80.
6. Aibinder WR, Izadpanah A, Elhassan BT. Ulnar shortening versus distal radius corrective osteotomy in the management of ulnar impaction after distal radius malunion. Hand (N Y) 2018;13(2):194–201.
7. Baek GH, Lee HJ, Gong HS, et al. Long-term outcomes of ulnar shortening osteotomy for idiopathic ulnar impaction syndrome: at least 5-years follow-up. Clin Orthop Surg 2011;3(4):295–301.
8. Milch H. Cuff resection of the ulna for malunited Colles' fracture. J Bone Joint Surg 1941;23(2):311–3.
9. Chen F, Osterman AL, Mahony K. Smoking and bony union after ulna-shortening osteotomy. Am J Orthop 2001;30(6):486–9.
10. Gaspar MP, Kane PM, Zohn RC, et al. Variables prognostic for delayed union and nonunion following ulnar shortening fixed with a dedicated osteotomy plate. J Hand Surg Am 2016;41(2):237–43.e1-e2.
11. Cha SM, Shin HD, Ahn KJ. Prognostic factors affecting union after ulnar shortening osteotomy in ulnar impaction syndrome: a retrospective case-control study. J Bone Joint Surg Am 2017;99(8): 638–47.
12. Gupta R, Bingenheimer E, Fornalski S, et al. The effect of ulnar shortening on lunate and triquetrum motion–a cadaveric study. Clin Biomech (Bristol, Avon) 2005;20(8):839–45.
13. Terzis A, Neubrech F, Sebald J, et al. Die Behandlung des ulnokarpalen Impaktionssyndroms. Handchirurgie Scan 2019;08(3):201–16.
14. Tolat AR, Stanley JK, Trail IA. A cadaveric study of the anatomy and stability of the distal radioulnar joint in the coronal and transverse planes. J Hand Surg Br 1996;21(5):587–94.
15. Prommersberger K-J, Kalb K, van Schoonhoven J. [Mal-united fractures of the distal radius–biomechanics and operative treatment options]. Handchir Mikrochir Plast Chir 2007;39(1):9–18.

16. Feldon P, Terrono AL, Belsky MR. The "wafer" procedure. Partial distal ulnar resection. Clin Orthop Relat Res 1992;275:124–9.

17. Oh W-T, Kang H-J, Chun Y-M, et al. Arthroscopic wafer procedure versus ulnar shortening osteotomy as a surgical treatment for idiopathic ulnar impaction syndrome. Arthroscopy 2018;34(2):421–30.

18. Meftah M, Keefer EP, Panagopoulos G, et al. Arthroscopic wafer resection for ulnar impaction syndrome: prediction of outcomes. Hand Surg 2010; 15(2):89–93.

19. Wnorowski DC, Palmer AK, Werner FW, et al. Anatomic and biomechanical analysis of the arthroscopic wafer procedure. Arthroscopy 1992;8(2): 204–12.

20. Del Gaudio T, Haerle M. Die arthroskopische ulnokarpale Dekompression durch Teilresektion des Ulnakopfs. Oper Orthop Traumatol 2016;28(4):263–9.

21. Bernstein MA, Nagle DJ, Martinez A, et al. A comparison of combined arthroscopic triangular fibrocartilage complex debridement and arthroscopic wafer distal ulna resection versus arthroscopic triangular fibrocartilage complex debridement and ulnar shortening osteotomy for ulnocarpal abutment syndrome. Arthroscopy 2004; 20(4):392–401.

22. Faber KJ, Iordache S, Grewal R. Magnetic resonance imaging for ulnar wrist pain. J Hand Surg Am 2010;35(2):303–7.

23. Constantine KJ, Tomaino MM, Herndon JH, et al. Comparison of ulnar shortening osteotomy and the wafer resection procedure as treatment for ulnar impaction syndrome. J Hand Surg Am 2000;25(1): 55–60.

24. Vandenberghe L, Degreef I, Didden K, et al. Ulnar shortening or arthroscopic wafer resection for ulnar impaction syndrome. Acta Orthop Belg 2012;78(3): 323–6.

25. Smet LD, Vandenberghe L, Degreef I. Ulnar impaction syndrome: ulnar shortening vs. arthroscopic wafer procedure. J Wrist Surg 2014;3(2):98–100.

26. Dailey SW, Palmer AK. The role of arthroscopy in the evaluation and treatment of triangular fibrocartilage complex injuries in athletes. Hand Clin 2000;16(3): 461–76.

27. Thurston AJ, Stanley JK. Hamato-lunate impingement: an uncommon cause of ulnar-sided wrist pain. Arthroscopy 2000;16(5):540–4.

28. Viegas SF, Wagner K, Patterson R, et al. Medial (hamate) facet of the lunate. J Hand Surg 1990; 15(4):564–71.

29. Yao J, Osterman AL. Arthroscopic techniques for wrist arthritis (radial styloidectomy and proximal pole hamate excisions). Hand Clin 2005;21(4): 519–26.

30. Viegas SF, Patterson RM, Hokanson JA, et al. Wrist anatomy: incidence, distribution, and correlation of anatomic variations, tears, and arthrosis. J Hand Surg 1993;18(3):463–75.

31. Harley BJ, Werner FW, Boles SD, et al. Arthroscopic resection of arthrosis of the proximal hamate: a clinical and biomechanical study. J Hand Surg Am 2004;29(4):661–7.

32. Slutsky DJ. Arthroscopic management of ulnocarpal impaction syndrome and ulnar styloid impaction syndrome. Hand Clin 2017;33(4):639–50.

33. Topper SM, Wood MB, Ruby LK. Ulnar styloid impaction syndrome. J Hand Surg Am 1997;22(4): 699–704.

34. Tomaino MM, Gainer M, Towers JD. Carpal impaction with the ulnar styloid process: treatment with partial styloid resection. J Hand Surg Br 2001; 26(3):252–5.

35. Bain GI, Bidwell TA. Arthroscopic excision of ulnar styloid in stylocarpal impaction. Arthroscopy 2006; 22(6):677.e1–3.

36. Giachino AA, McIntyre AI, Guy KJ, et al. Ulnar styloid triquetral impaction. Hand Surg 2007;12(2): 123–34.

37. Sauerbier M, Eisenschenk A, Krimmer H, et al. Die Handchirurgie. München, Germany: Urban & Fischer Verlag/Elsevier GmbH; 2014.

Distal Radioulnar Joint Instability

Brandon Boyd, MD[a], Julie Adams, MD[b],*

KEYWORDS

- Distal radioulnar joint • DRUJ • DRUJ Instability • Triangular fibrocartilage complex • TFCC

KEY POINTS

- The distal radioulnar joint (DRUJ) is an inherently unstable joint relying heavily on the surrounding soft tissues to maintain function and stability.
- Instability to the DRUJ can occur secondary to osseous injuries and/or soft tissue injuries.
- Acute instability most commonly occurs in conjunction with a concomitant fracture of the radius or distal ulna but can also occur as an isolated dislocation of the DRUJ.
- Chronic instability is a result of a history of injury leading to articular incongruity of the DRUJ, injury to the TFCC, or a combination of both.
- Treatment of acute injuries involves anatomic reduction of the DRUJ with or without TFCC repair and a period of immobilization.
- Treatment of chronic injuries requires correcting any underlying osseous deformity and subsequent repair or reconstruction of the TFCC.

INTRODUCTION

Instability of the distal radioulnar joint (DRUJ) is a source of ulnar-sided wrist pain and functional impairment. Symptomatic instability may present acutely, after a recent traumatic injury, or in a delayed fashion as chronic instability following a history of a traumatic event. Instability of the DRUJ is dorsal or palmar, multidirectional, and/or proximal-distal (or forearm longitudinal) instability, as seen with an Essex-Lopresti type injury. A detailed understanding of the complex anatomy, biomechanics, and stabilizing structures of the DRUJ is important to evaluate and treat acute and chronic instability. This article provides a review of the relevant anatomy, and the clinical assessment and management of conditions leading to DRUJ instability.

ANATOMY

The DRUJ is a diarthrodial synovial articulation that functions to transmit loads from the ulnar carpus to the ulna and to allow for wrist motion and forearm rotation.[1] Although by convention "ulnar" variance is talked about with ulnar-positive or ulnar-negative variance, the ulna is the fixed unit in the forearm around which the radius rotates at the proximal radioulnar joint and the DRUJ. The inherent bony stability to the DRUJ is minimal because of the radius of curvature mismatch between the sigmoid notch of the distal radius and the ulnar head. The average radius of curvature of the sigmoid notch is 15 to 19 mm compared with only 10 mm for the ulnar head.[2] Therefore, DRUJ stability is highly reliant on the static and dynamic soft tissue stabilizers surrounding the joint. The dynamic structures

[a] Hand and Upper Extremity Fellow, Philadelphia Hand to Shoulder Center, 834 Chestnut Street, G114, Philadelphia, PA 19107, USA; [b] Department of Orthopaedic Surgery, University of Tennessee College of Medicine-Chattanooga, 960 East Third Street, Suite 100, Chattanooga, TN 37403, USA
* Corresponding author.
E-mail address: adams.julie.e@gmail.com

Hand Clin 37 (2021) 563–573
https://doi.org/10.1016/j.hcl.2021.06.011

that contribute to DRUJ stability are the pronator quadratus and extensor carpi ulnaris (ECU) muscles, but these are believed to be less important than the static stabilizers. Static stabilizing structures include the DRUJ capsule, interosseous membrane (IOM), and the triangular fibrocartilage complex (TFCC).[3] The TFCC is arguably the most important set of structures for maintaining normal DRUJ kinematics.[4,5] It is composed of the dorsal and volar radioulnar ligaments, ulnolunate ligament, ulnotriquetral ligament, meniscal homologue, central articular disk, and the subsheath of the ECU tendon (**Fig. 1**). These structures combine to provide load-bearing and load-sharing functions for the ulnocarpal joint and soft tissue stabilization of the DRUJ.

The dorsal and volar radioulnar ligaments are the most important components, of the TFCC, responsible for stability of the DRUJ. The dorsal and volar ligaments extend from the dorsal and volar margins of the sigmoid notch and subsequently divide, in the coronal plane, into two separate limbs. The superficial limbs insert into the midportion of the ulnar styloid, whereas the deep limbs, also referred to as the ligamentum subcruentum, insert into the fovea of the distal ulna (**Fig. 2**). During forearm protonation the dorsal deep and volar superficial fibers tighten, whereas with forearm supination the dorsal superficial and volar deep fibers tighten to provide DRUJ stability.[3,6,7]

The articular disk is surrounded volarly and dorsally by the radioulnar ligaments and is responsible for load transmission of the ulnocarpal joint. However, the articular disk has a minimal role in providing stability to the DRUJ. The ulnolunate and ulnotriquetral ligaments represent volar thickenings of the capsule and originate from the volar radioulnar ligament and articular disk and insert distally on the lunate and triquetrum, respectively.[8] These ligaments connect the ulna to the carpus through the palmar foveal insertion of the radioulnar ligament.[8] In addition, the ulnolunate and ulnotriquetral ligaments assist in preventing excessive dorsal translation of the distal ulna relative to the carpus.

The meniscal homologue is a loose connective tissue structure that runs between the ulnocarpal capsule, articular disk, and proximal aspect of the triquetrum.[2,9] It has insertions onto the triquetrum and a broader insertion onto the fifth metacarpal.[2,9] Although the exact role of this structure is not known, it does not provide a significant structural stability to the DRUJ. The ECU subsheath, located at the floor of the sixth dorsal extensor compartment, extends from the dorsal radioulnar ligament to the carpus. It provides

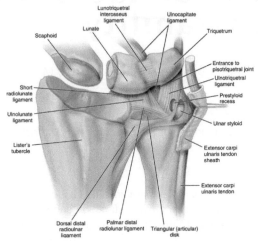

Fig. 1. Anatomy of the triangular fibrocartilage complex and associated structures. (*From* Kovachevich R, Elhassan BT. Arthroscopic and open repair of the TFCC. Hand Clin. 2010;26(4):485-494. doi:10.1016/j.hcl.2010.07.003; with permission)

reinforcement to the dorsal capsule separate from the dynamic stabilizing effect from the ECU.[2,8]

In addition to the TFCC, the IOM not only provides stability to the forearm as a unit but also plays a role in stabilizing the DRUJ. Noda and colleagues[10] identified the distal oblique bundle, which

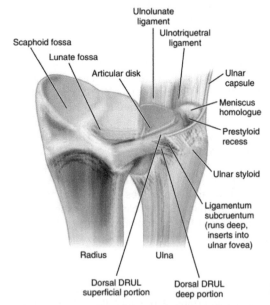

Fig. 2. Anatomy of the foveal attachment of the triangular fibrocartilage complex and the ligamentum subcruentum. DRUL, distal radioulnar ligament. (*From* Ko JH, Wiedrich TA. Triangular fibrocartilage complex injuries in the elite athlete. Hand Clin. 2012;28(3):307-viii. doi:10.1016/j.hcl.2012.05.014; with permission)

originates from the distal one-sixth of the ulnar shaft and runs distally to insert on the inferior rim of the sigmoid notch (**Fig. 3**). The presence of the distal oblique bundle acts as a secondary stabilizer to the DRUJ, especially when the volar and dorsal radioulnar ligaments have been injured.[3,10,11]

HISTORY

Although frequently history is straightforward, particularly in the setting of an acute injury, patients may not articulate or appreciate instability as such. Important aspects of the patient's history should include detailed information regarding traumatic events, age, hand dominance, occupational demands, and recreational activities. Information regarding the history of injuries, and subsequent treatments, should be obtained in patients presenting with chronic complaints. Specific aspects of the history are reviewed later for acute and chronic DRUJ instability in their respective sections.

PHYSICAL EXAMINATION

The physical examination generally begins with an overall inspection of the affected extremity. The examiner should inspect for any skin lesions, scars, swelling, and/or deformities and use the contralateral extremity for comparison. The wrist can then be palpated to examine for any localized areas of tenderness. Active and passive range of motion of the wrist and forearm should be assessed for flexion-extension, radial-ulnar deviation, and pronation-supination and compared with contralateral extremity. A detailed motor and sensory examination should be performed and documented, in addition to vascular status. Following this comprehensive assessment, there are multiple provocative tests that can help the examiner diagnose the pathology and formulate a treatment plan. We review more specific physical examination findings and tests in each section that follows.

IMAGING
Radiographs

Initial imaging evaluation should begin with plain film radiographs to include standard posteroanterior (PA), oblique, and lateral radiographs of the wrist and in some cases, standard two-view radiographs of the forearm and possibly the elbow. Certain plain film findings raise suspicion of possible DRUJ instability. On the PA or anteroposterior (AP) view of the wrist, a widened space between the radius and ulna is indicative of instability; alternatively, a dislocated DRUJ may be visualized with lack of contour and visualization of overlap of the radius and ulna. The lateral film should be critically assessed to visualize that the radius and ulna are in the same plane; if the two bones are divergent on a true lateral, instability may be present.[12] In the setting of distal radius fractures, a translational gap between the radius and ulna is highly predictive of instability as outlined by Fujitani and colleagues.[13] An ulnar styloid fracture involving the base and/or with displacement of greater than 2 mm has been shown to be a risk factor for DRUJ instability associated with distal radius fractures, although other series fail to identify styloid fractures as a marker for instability.[13,14]

In addition to bony abnormalities, ulnar-positive variance may alert the clinician of possible DRUJ instability. Shen and colleagues[15] suggested that

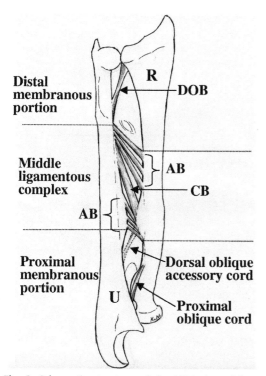

Fig. 3. Schematic structure of the IOM viewed from the anterior aspect of a right forearm. IOM consists of distal, middle, and proximal portions. Middle portion is a ligamentous complex further divided into the central band (CB) and the accessory band (AB). The distal oblique bundle (DOB) originates from the distal one-sixth of the ulnar shaft and runs distally to insert on the inferior rim of the sigmoid notch. (*From* Noda K, Goto A, Murase T, Sugamoto K, Yoshikawa H, Moritomo H. Interosseous membrane of the forearm: an anatomical study of ligament attachment locations. J Hand Surg Am. 2009;34(3):415-422. doi:10.1016/j.jhsa.2008.10.025; with permission)

a traumatic injury to the TFCC with radiographic evidence of ulnar-positive variance, greater than the asymptomatic side, may be an indication of disruption of the deep radioulnar ligaments. Stress radiographs may also be helpful in diagnosing DRUJ instability, especially in patients with chronic instability. Iida and colleagues[16] found that DRUJ widening and increased gap distance with clenched-fist PA stress views was significantly greater in injured wrists than contralateral normal wrists.

Computed Tomography

Computed tomography (CT) scans are useful to evaluate fracture patterns, malunions, deformities of ulnar head or sigmoid notch, and joint reduction and congruency. In the acute setting CT is more commonly used to assess fracture pattern, with bony injuries, and/or the DRUJ joint reduction and congruency following reduction of an acutely subluxated or dislocated DRUJ. However, CT scan is also helpful for evaluating DRUJ instability in the chronic setting. The axial cuts on CT scan are especially helpful for evaluating joint congruency and are performed with the forearm in protonation, neutral, and supination. It may also be useful to image the contralateral wrist at the same time to detect subtle incongruencies and instabilities. Multiple methods for measuring DRUJ instability have been described and include the use of dorsal and palmar radioulnar lines as described by Mino and colleagues, the epicenter method and congruency method as described by Wechsler and colleagues, and more recently the radioulnar ratio described by Lo and colleagues.[3,17–19] Lo and colleagues[17] believed the Mino and Wechsler methods underestimated and overestimated the extent of DRUJ subluxation. Therefore, they described the radioulnar ratio to identify DRUJ instability. This involves finding the center of the ulnar head (C) using concentric circles and a line connecting the volar (A) and dorsal (B) margins of the sigmoid notch. A second line drawn perpendicular to line AB is then drawn to the center of the ulnar head (line CD).[17] The ratio of length AD/AB is then calculated (**Fig. 4**). The authors found the radioulnar ratio was able to detect subluxation earlier than the other described methods and may be a more sensitive tool for detecting subtle instability.[17] However, there is still no gold standard in diagnosing instability using CT scans. Therefore, imaging both wrists in protonation, supination, and neutral should be strongly considered and correlating CT findings with physical examination findings to help accurately diagnose DRUJ instability.

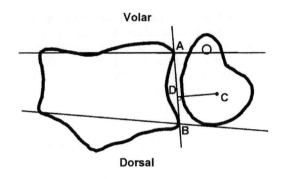

$$\text{Normal RUR} = \frac{AD}{AB} \pm 2\,SD$$

Fig. 4. RUR method. The center of the ulnar head is found using concentric circles. A line similar to that used in the epicenter method is drawn from the dorsal and volar margins of the sigmoid notch. A line perpendicular to this line is drawn to the center of the ulnar head. The AD/AB ratio is the RUR. RUR, radioulnar ratio. (*From* Lo IK, MacDermid JC, Bennett JD, Bogoch E, King GJ. The radioulnar ratio: a new method of quantifying distal radioulnar joint subluxation. J Hand Surg Am. 2001;26(2):236-243. doi:10.1053/jhsu.2001.22908; with permission)

MRI

MRI is a highly sensitive and specific imaging modality for evaluating the TFCC and DRUJ. Ideally, MRI of the wrist would be performed with a dedicated wrist coil in a 3.0-T scanner, compared with a 1.5-T scanner, because this improves the capability for detection of TFCC injuries (**Fig. 5**).[20] In addition to identifying TFCC tears, Ehman and colleagues[21] found that ulnar head subluxation in relation to the sigmoid notch of the radius is a good predictor of tears at the foveal attachment of the volar and dorsal radioulnar ligaments.

ACUTE INSTABILITY OF THE DISTAL RADIOULNAR JOINT
Isolated Distal Radioulnar Joint Dislocations

Evaluation
Isolated DRUJ dislocations generally occur less frequently than DRUJ dislocations associated with a concomitant forearm fracture.[12,22] However, when isolated dislocations occur, they are either dorsal or volar, with dorsal being more common. Dorsal dislocations are thought to occur with forced hyperpronation of the wrist/forearm, such as with a fall onto an outstretched hand.[23] Patients generally present with their forearm fixed in protonation with an inability to supinate and a prominent dorsal ulna at the wrist.[12] Conversely, volar

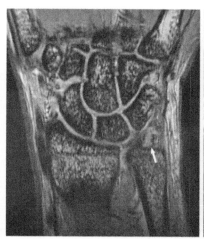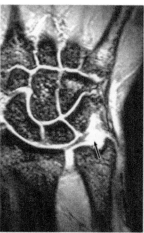

Fig. 5. MRI coronal cuts showing a Palmer class 1B TFCC tear. Note the loss of the low signal of the TFCC at the foveal attachment (*white arrow*) in the image on the right, with the concomitant high signal intensity at the region of the fovea (*black arrow*). (*From* Nakamura T, Sato K, Okazaki M, Toyama Y, Ikegami H. Repair of foveal detachment of the triangular fibrocartilage complex: open and arthroscopic transosseous techniques. Hand Clin. 2011;27(3):281-290. doi:10.1016/j.hcl.2011.05.002; with permission)

dislocations of the DRUJ occur because of a hypersupination force and present with the forearm locked in supination with the inability to pronate.

Initial plain film imaging should consist of two views of the wrist, forearm, and elbow. With an acute DRUJ dislocation, the AP view may reveal widening of the DRUJ and divergence of the distal radius and ulna in a dorsal dislocation and overlap of the distal radius and ulna in a volar dislocation.[12]

Management

Management begins with attempted closed reduction in the emergency department with local anesthesia and/or conscious sedation. Dorsal dislocations should be reduced with longitudinal traction, recreating the deformity with protonation and subsequent dorsal pressure over the ulnar head followed by supinating the wrist. With volar dislocations, the examiner should again apply longitudinal traction, hypersupinate the wrist, and apply volar pressure to the ulnar head with subsequent protonation of the wrist to achieve reduction. Reductions are visualized on clinical examination with a palpable clunk and restoration of the normal appearance of the wrist. However, reductions should be confirmed with plain film imaging and the stability of the wrist should be examined with the forearm in neutral, protonation, and supination. Generally, the wrist is most stable in supination with dorsal dislocations, and in protonation with volar dislocations.[12] Once reduced, the forearm and wrist should be immobilized in the position with maximal stability to the DRUJ. Immobilization should be continued for 6 weeks. If the DRUJ remains grossly unstable following closed reduction, the surgeon should first confirm that reduction is truly adequate, and that there is no soft tissue

interposition prohibiting reduction. Once this is confirmed, the surgeon needs to consider stabilization of the DRUJ. This may take the form of a TFCC repair, fixation of an ulnar styloid fracture, or pinning of the DRUJ in a reduced position. Two ulnarly to radially directed 0.062-inch K-wires are introduced from the ulnar aspect of the wrist proximal to the DRUJ. Pins will cross four cortices (at the ulna and radius) to exit the radial cortex of the radius, such that retrieval is possible should the pins break. Our preference is to have the pins just extrude from the radial cortex to avoid irritation of the superficial radial nerve. Typically, the forearm is positioned in supination, for dorsal dislocations, or protonation, for volar dislocations. The forearm and wrist should be immobilized in a sugar tong or Muenster cast or splint with pins in place for 6 weeks.

If closed reduction maneuvers fail, soft tissue interposition precluding the reduction of the DRUJ is likely the cause. Open reduction is required to remove the interposing soft tissue structures. Before open reduction, obtaining advanced imaging, such as an MRI or more rarely, CT scan, is beneficial to gain further information regarding potential blocks to reduction. Several mechanisms for irreducible DRUJ dislocations have been described and include the ECU, extensor digitorum communis to ring and long fingers, fragments of a torn TFCC, impaction fracture of the ulna on the sigmoid notch, and the median nerve.[24–28] Open reduction is typically performed through a dorsal approach overlying the fifth dorsal extensor compartment. Following removal of interposing structures, repair of the TFCC and/or pinning of the radius and ulna just proximal to the DRUJ with two 0.062-inch K-wires is performed for additional stability (**Figs. 6** and **7**). A

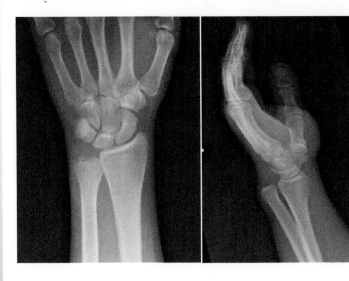

Fig. 6. PA and lateral radiograph of an L wrist with an acute open dorsal dislocation of the DRUJ. Note the small associated ulnar styloid fracture on the PA, and the overlap of the radius and ulna even on a good PA view, indicative of dislocation. Patient had unsuccessful closed reduction in the emergency department and subsequently went to the operating room for irrigation and debridement, removal of the interposed ECU tendon, repair of the TFCC, and pinning of the DRUJ in supination.

sugar tong splint is applied in the operating room and then transitioned to a Muenster cast for 6 weeks postoperatively.

Fractures Associated with Distal Radioulnar Joint Instability

Evaluation
Acute injury to the DRUJ most commonly occurs in association with concomitant forearm fractures including distal radius fractures, radial shaft fractures, distal ulnar/ulnar styloid fractures, and Essex-Lopresti injuries.

Distal radius fractures are common and represent approximately 3% of all upper extremity injuries with incidence of more than 640,000 in the United States annually.[29] Associated injuries to the TFCC with distal radius fractures may be 60% to 84%; however, most of these do not result in DRUJ instability.[30,31] Patients with injuries and associated DRUJ instability do have worse functional outcomes after a median follow-up of 12 months.[31]

Essex-Lopresti injuries involve fracture of the radial head/neck with subsequent disruption of the IOM and DRUJ. As with most DRUJ injuries, the instability pattern is typically in a dorsal direction, but because of the injury to the longitudinal stabilizing structures, patients may have overt

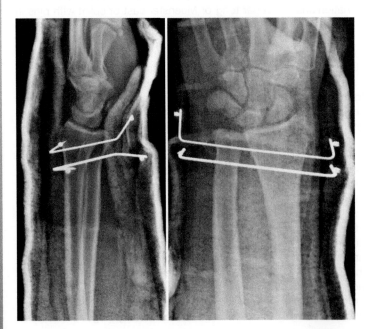

Fig. 7. PA and lateral views of L wrist postoperatively status post open reduction and pinning of the DRUJ with two 0.062-inch K-wires in supination. Our preference is generally to pass the K-wires from ulnar to radial, and have just the tips extrude from the radial cortex to avoid injury to the superficial radial nerve. The pins are typically cut and buried under the skin for later retrieval via the ulnar side of the forearm.

ulnar-positive variance without dorsal or volar translation. Galeazzi fractures involve a radial shaft fracture with associated injury and instability in the DRUJ. Initial evaluation of these injuries is similar to that previously described for isolated acute DRUJ dislocations.

Management

Initial management of operative distal radius and radial shaft fractures should include open reduction and internal fixation followed by assessment of the DRUJ. An adequate preoperative evaluation of the contralateral forearm and wrist is helpful in assessing the amount of physiologic motion present in the uninjured DRUJ. Some authors have suggested that greater than 1 cm of dorsal to palmar translation signifies instability.[32] If the patient's DRUJ is reduced but is unstable, then stability of the DRUJ is checked in positions of forearm pronation, supination, or neutral. If the wrist is globally unstable, then the DRUJ is stabilized, by fixation of an ulnar styloid fracture, TFCC repair, or pinning the DRUJ in a reduced posture for 6 weeks. If, however, a stable position can be found in a given position of forearm rotation (usually supination), then the forearm is immobilized in the position of maximal stability for 6 weeks following surgery. Immobilization is performed in supination for dorsal instability and pronation for volar instability. In the known or suspected Essex-Lopresti injury, the radial head/neck is repaired anatomically, if possible (which it usually is not), otherwise a radial head replacement is performed. If the radial head is to be excised, one can evaluate the status of the injured forearm/wrist structures by the radial pull test.[33,34] The radial neck is grasped and pulled longitudinally, while fluoroscopy of the PA or AP wrist is performed to evaluate the change in ulnar variance. This can help document and diagnose injury to the DRUJ/TFCC and the IOM. Following assessment and treatment of the elbow, the wrist is assessed for stability by the pull test and clinical examination in pronation, supination, and neutral. If the DRUJ is unstable, a TFCC repair is generally undertaken and the forearm is immobilized. If the IOM is injured, treatment is a matter of discussion. Typically, these are midsubstance tears and not primarily repairable; augmentation with suture button constructs, allograft or autograft tendon or bone tendon bone, or tendon transfer from the pronator have been described.[35–38]

CHRONIC INSTABILITY OF THE DISTAL RADIOULNAR JOINT

In patients presenting with chronic instability of the DRUJ, the cause may be articular incongruity,

ligamentous disruption, or a combination of both.[39] The history is an important place to begin to identify a history of traumatic injury and subsequent treatment or lack thereof. There may be a history of a distal radius fracture, a DRUJ dislocation event in the past, or simply a fall on an outstretched hand. Patients typically complain of ulnar-sided wrist pain, loss of forearm rotation, and possible clunking sensation, especially with activities related to protonation and supination of the wrist and forearm. Left untreated, DRUJ instability can lead to functional impairment because of pain, decreased grip strength, and arthritis.[40]

Evaluation

Physical examination should begin with inspection of the affected wrist and compared with the contralateral extremity to look for asymmetries related to the resting posture of the forearm and wrist. Palpation for localized areas of tenderness should then be performed. The ulnar fovea sign is performed by palpating the area between the ulnar styloid and the flexor carpi ulnaris tendon.[41] Pain associated with this test is sensitive and specific for a foveal tear of the radioulnar ligaments or an ulnotriquetral ligament tear.[41] The DRUJ shuck test is performed by holding the distal radius with the thumb and index finger of one hand and the distal ulna by the index and thumb of contralateral hand and testing the amount of AP translation between the radius and ulna with forearm in neutral, protonation, and supination. Increased translation compared with the contralateral extremity is a sign of DRUJ instability. The piano key sign is performed with the forearm in full protonation with palmar depression of the ulnar head and then subsequent release of the pressure on the dorsal aspect of the ulnar head. The test is considered positive if pain is elicited following release of pressure on the ulnar head.[2,42]

Initial plain film imaging should be obtained to look for distal radius fracture malunions, DRUJ widening, subluxation of the ulna volarly or dorsally in relation to the sigmoid notch, and/or presence of DRUJ arthritis. CT scans may be beneficial to further evaluate the alignment of the distal radius and the sigmoid notch in the setting of a malunion. It may also be helpful to confirm subtle instability, noted on clinical examination, by the methods previously described after obtaining scans of the affected and unaffected wrists in neutral, protonation, and supination. MRI may be helpful to evaluate the status of the soft tissue stabilizers.

Management

Although most commonly we offer immediate surgical management for DRUJ instability, nonoperative treatment is an option particularly for elderly or infirm patients in whom symptoms do not rise to a level of much concern. Concern regarding nonoperative treatment includes the expectation that asymmetric wear of the cartilage at the DRUJ will predictably lead to arthritis. Patients who choose nonoperative care should be advised of this. In those who choose nonoperative care, treatment is aimed at reducing painful symptoms with activity modifications, nonsteroidal anti-inflammatory drugs, corticosteroid injections, and stabilization bracing (**Fig. 8**). Millard and colleagues[43,44] found that prefabricated and custom braces help reduce DRUJ instability in full protonation and supination.

In almost all cases, surgical intervention is the preferred option for patients to ameliorate pain, loss of motion, and loss of function because of instability. Contraindications to TFCC repair versus reconstruction include ulnocarpal impaction and length discrepancies between the radius and ulna, inflammatory arthritis, and osteoarthritis of the DRUJ.[40] Patients that present with instability associated with distal radius malunion may be candidates for corrective osteotomy of the radius and subsequent TFCC repair or reconstruction if instability remains following correction of the malunion. TFCC repair is attempted if the soft tissues are amenable. However, when the TFCC is irreparable, but DRUJ arthrosis is not

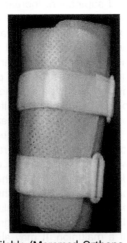

Fig. 8. A commercially available (Maramed Orthopedic Systems, Hialeah, FL) prefabricated forearm brace (*left*). A custom forearm brace (*right*). (*From* Millard GM, Budoff JE, Paravic V, Noble PC. Functional bracing for distal radioulnar joint instability. J Hand Surg Am. 2002;27(6):972-977. doi:10.1053/jhsu.2002.36542; with permission)

problematic, a reconstructive stabilization procedure is performed.

When the TFCC is repairable, our preference is to perform an open repair, although recent techniques highlighting arthroscopic bony repairs represent an alternative with reported good results. Arthroscopy may be performed initially as a diagnostic tool, but then an open incision is made. If performing a malunion correction of the distal radius, then correcting the distal radius deformity is performed initially followed by open repair or reconstruction of the TFCC. A longitudinal incision is then made over the fifth extensor compartment, which is then opened and released. An "L"-shaped capsulotomy is made, with one limb proximal and parallel do the dorsal radioulnar ligament and the second limb along the sigmoid notch (**Fig. 9**). A braided slowly absorbable suture or Prolene or PDS suture is passed in a horizontal mattress fashion through the TFCC, then through holes drilled up into the foveal region and tied over the ulnar neck. Keith needles loaded on a mini-driver to pass through the bone facilitates passage of the sutures. The capsulotomy is then repaired anatomically and the forearm and wrist are splinted with a sugar tong splint in supination for dorsal instability and protonation for volar instability. The splint is then transitioned to a Muenster cast at the 2-week postoperative appointment for an additional 4 weeks. Patients then begin a progressive range of motion and strengthening program with anticipated return to unrestricted activities by 3 months postoperatively.

In cases where the TFCC is irreparable, a reconstructive procedure is chosen. There are several techniques used for TFCC reconstruction including a distally based strip of the ECU tendon through the TFCC.[45] More commonly, use of a palmaris longus graft (or a strip of the flexor carpi ulnaris if the palmaris longus is absent) is performed to reconstruct the distal radioulnar ligaments.[46] The approach and capsulotomy are performed as described previously through the fifth extensor compartment. The distal radius is then exposed by elevating the fourth extensor compartment subperiosteally such that an area of 5 mm proximal to the radiolunate joint and 5 mm radial to the sigmoid notch is revealed. A K-wire is then placed at this site from dorsal to volar and overdrilled with a 3.5-mm cannulated drill bit. A longitudinal volar-based incision is made just radial to the ulnar neurovascular bundle and a second tunnel site is identified from the fovea at the base of the ulnar styloid to the metaphyseal ulnar neck region. A K-wire is then passed from the fovea out ulnarly and proximally and a cannulated 3.5-mm drill bit is used to overdrill this site. The tendon graft

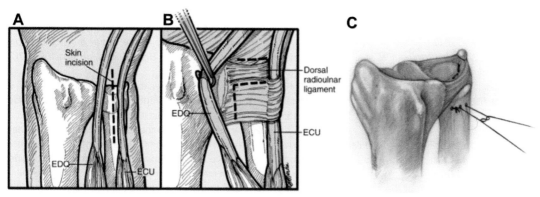

Fig. 9. (*A–C*) Open approach through the fifth extensor compartment and an "L"-shaped capsulotomy to expose the DRUJ and proximal surface of the TFCC. A second horizontal incision can be made parallel and just distal to the dorsal radioulnar ligaments to visualize the distal surface of the TFCC and pass sutures. Horizontal mattress sutures are passed through the TFCC and then tied over bone tunnels exiting through the ulnar neck. EDQ, extensor digiti quinti. (*From* Adams BD, Leversedge FJ. Green's Operative Hand Surgery: Distal Radioulnar Joint. 7th Edition. Philadelphia, PA: Elsevier; 2017. Copyright Elizabeth Martin; with permission)

is then passed from volar to dorsal and retrieved (**Fig. 10**). A hemostat is then passed from dorsal to volar over the ulnar head and proximal to the TFCC, exiting through the volar DRUJ capsule to grasp and retrieve the tendon graft, which is pulled into the dorsal wound. The two limbs of the graft are then passed through the ulnar tunnel to exit at the ulnar border of the forearm. The two limbs are crossed and then passed in opposite directions around the ulnar neck with the more dorsal limb placed under the ECU. With compression of the DRUJ and tensioning in neutral rotation, the two limbs are tied to each other and sutured in place. The capsulotomy is then closed and the extensor digiti minimi (EDM) is left out of its retinacular sheath. The forearm and wrist are splinted with a sugar tong splint in supination for dorsal instability and protonation for volar instability. The splint is

then transitioned to a Muenster cast at the 2-week postoperative appointment for an additional 4 weeks. Patients then begin a progressive range of motion and strengthening program with anticipated return to unrestricted activities by 3 months postoperatively.

When DRUJ instability presents in the setting of arthrosis, salvage procedures are an option, as described elsewhere in this issue.

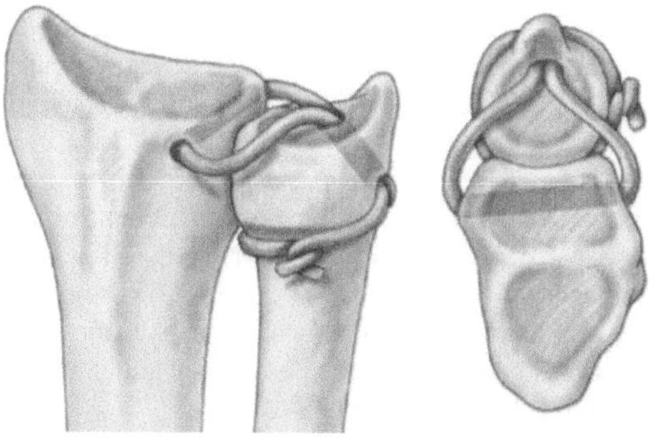

CLINICS CARE POINTS

- The distal radioulnar joint (DRUJ) is an inherently unstable joint relying heavily on the surrounding soft tissues to maintain function and stability.
- The triangular fibrocartilage complex (TFCC) is composed of the dorsal and volar radioulnar ligaments, an articular disk, meniscal homologue, ulnolunate ligament, ulnotriquetral ligaments, and the extensor carpi ulnaris (ECU) subsheath.
- Instability to the DRUJ can occur secondary to osseous injuries and/or soft tissue injuries.
- Acute instability most commonly occurs in conjunction with a concomitant fracture of the radius.

Fig. 10. Tendon graft reconstruction to stabilize the distal radioulnar joint. (*From* Lawler E, Adams BD. Reconstruction for DRUJ instability. Hand (N Y). 2007;2(3):123-126.   doi:10.1007/s11552-007-9034-6; with permission)

REFERENCES

1. Chu-Kay Mak M, Ho PC. Arthroscopic-assisted triangular fibrocartilage complex reconstruction. Hand Clin 2017;33(4):625–37.

2. Adams BD, Leversedge FJ. Green's operative hand surgery: distal radioulnar joint. 7th ed. Philadelphia (PA): Elsevier; 2017.

3. Kihara H, Short WH, Werner FW, et al. The stabilizing mechanism of the distal radioulnar joint during pronation and supination. J Hand Surg Am 1995;20:930–6.

4. Adams BD, Lawler E. Chronic instability of the distal radioulnar joint. J Am Acad Orthop Surg 2007;15: 571–5.

5. Palmer AK, Werner FW. The triangular fibrocartilage complex of the wrist: anatomy and function. J Hand Surg Am 1981;6:153–62.

6. Kleinman WB. Stability of the distal radioulna joint: biomechanics, pathophysiology, physical diagnosis, and restoration of function what we have learned in 25 years. J Hand Surg Am 2007;32(7):1086–106.

7. Stuart PR, Berger RA, Linscheid RL, et al. The dorsopalmar stability of the distal radioulnar joint. J Hand Surg Am 2000;25(4):689–99.

8. Nakamura T, Takayama S, Horiuchi Y, et al. Origins and insertions of the triangular fibrocartilage complex: a histological study. J Hand Surg Br 2001; 26(5):446–54.

9. Nishikawa S, Toh S. Anatomical study of the carpal attachment of the triangular fibrocartilage complex. J Bone Joint Surg Br 2002;84(7):1062–5.

10. Noda K, Goto A, Murase T, et al. Interosseous membrane of the forearm: an anatomical study of ligament attachment locations. J Hand Surg Am 2009; 34(3):415–22.

11. Kitamura T, Moritomo H, Arimitsu S, et al. The biomechanical effect of the distal interosseous membrane on distal radioulnar joint stability: a preliminary anatomic study. J Hand Surg Am 2011;36(10): 1626–30.

12. Carlsen BT, Dennison DG, Moran SL. Acute dislocations of the distal radioulnar joint and distal ulna fractures. Hand Clin 2010;26(4):503–16.

13. Fujitani R, Omokawa S, Akahane M, et al. Predictors of distal radioulnar joint instability in distal radius fractures. J Hand Surg Am 2011;36(12):1919–25.

14. May MM, Lawton JN, Blazar PE. Ulnar styloid fractures associated with distal radius fractures: incidence and implications for distal radioulnar joint instability. J Hand Surg Am 2002;27(6):965–71.

15. Shen J, Papadonikolakis A, Garrett JP, et al. Ulnar-positive variance as a predictor of distal radioulnar joint ligament disruption. J Hand Surg Am 2005; 30(6):1172–7.

16. Iida A, Omokawa S, Akahane M, et al. Distal radioulnar joint stress radiography for detecting radioulnar ligament injury. J Hand Surg Am 2012;37(5):968–74.

17. Lo IK, MacDermid JC, Bennett JD, et al. The radioulnar ratio: a new method of quantifying distal radioulnar joint subluxation. J Hand Surg Am 2001;26(2): 236–43.

18. Mino DE, Palmer AK, Levinsohn EM. Radiography and computerized tomography in the diagnosis of incongruity of the distal radio-ulnar joint. A prospective study. J Bone Joint Surg Am 1985;67(2): 247–52.

19. Wechsler RJ, Wehbe MA, Rifkin MD, et al. Computed tomography diagnosis of distal radioulnar subluxation. Skeletal Radiol 1987;16(1):1–5.

20. Anderson ML, Skinner JA, Felmlee JP, et al. Diagnostic comparison of 1.5 Tesla and 3.0 Tesla preoperative MRI of the wrist in patients with ulnar-sided wrist pain. J Hand Surg Am 2008;33(7):1153–9.

21. Ehman EC, Hayes ML, Berger RA, et al. Subluxation of the distal radioulnar joint as a predictor of foveal triangular fibrocartilage complex tears. J Hand Surg Am 2011;36(11):1780–4.

22. Mikic ZD. Treatment of acute injuries of the triangular fibrocartilage complex associated with distal radioulnar joint instability. J Hand Surg Am 1995;20(2): 319–23.

23. Chidgey LK. The distal radioulnar joint: problems and solutions. J Am Acad Orthop Surg 1995;3(2): 95–109.

24. Bruckner JD, Alexander AH, Lichtman DM. Acute dislocations of the distal radioulnar joint. Instr Course Lect 1996;45:27–36.

25. Garrigues GE, Aldridge JM 3rd. Acute irreducible distal radioulnar joint dislocation. A case report. J Bone Joint Surg Am 2007;89(7):1594–7.

26. Itoh Y, Horiuchi Y, Takahashi M, et al. Extensor tendon involvement in Smith's and Galeazzi's fractures. J Hand Surg Am 1987;12(4):535–40.

27. Jenkins NH, Mintowt-Czyz WJ, Fairclough JA. Irreducible dislocation of the distal radioulnar joint. Injury 1987;18(1):40–3.

28. Paley D, Rubenstein J, McMurtry RY. Irreducible dislocation of distal radial ulnar joint. Orthop Rev 1986;15(4):228–31.

29. Chung KC, Spilson SV. The frequency and epidemiology of hand and forearm fractures in the United States. J Hand Surg Am 2001;26(5):908–15.

30. Geissler WB, Freeland AE, Savoie FH, et al. Intracarpal soft-tissue lesions associated with an intra-articular fracture of the distal end of the radius. J Bone Joint Surg Am 1996;78(3):357–65.

31. Lindau T, Adlercreutz C, Aspenberg P. Peripheral tears of the triangular fibrocartilage complex cause distal radioulnar joint instability after distal radial fractures. J Hand Surg Am 2000;25(3):464–8.

32. Ruch DS, Weiland AJ, Wolfe SW, et al. Current concepts in the treatment of distal radial fractures. Instr Course Lect 2004;53:389–401.

33. Kachooei AR, Rivlin M, Shojaie B, et al. Intraoperative technique for evaluation of the interosseous ligament of the forearm. J Hand Surg Am 2015;40(12): 2372–6.e1.

34. Smith AM, Urbanosky LR, Castle JA, et al. Radius pull test: predictor of longitudinal forearm instability. J Bone Joint Surg Am 2002;84(11):1970–6.

35. Adams JE, Osterman AL. The Essex-Lopresti injury: evaluation and treatment considerations. Hand Clin 2020;36(4):463–8.

36. Gaspar MP, Kane PM, Pflug EM, et al. Interosseous membrane reconstruction with a suture-button construct for treatment of chronic forearm instability. J Shoulder Elbow Surg 2016;25(9):1491–500.

37. Gaspar MP, Adams JE, Zohn RC, et al. Late reconstruction of the interosseous membrane with bone-patellar tendon-bone graft for chronic Essex-Lopresti injuries: outcomes with a mean follow-up of over 10 years. J Bone Joint Surg Am 2018;100(5):416–27.

38. Ruch DS, Chang DS, Koman LA. Reconstruction of longitudinal stability of the forearm after disruption of interosseous ligament and radial head excision (Essex-Lopresti lesion). J South Orthop Assoc 1999;8(1):47–52.

39. Faucher GK, Zimmerman RM, Zimmerman NB. Instability and arthritis of the distal radioulnar joint: a critical analysis review. JBJS Rev 2016;4(12).

https://doi.org/10.2106/JBJS.RVW.16.00005. 01874474-201612000-00001.

40. Kakar S, Carlsen BT, Moran SL, et al. The management of chronic distal radioulnar instability. Hand Clin 2010;26(4):517–28.

41. Tay SC, Tomita K, Berger RA. The "ulnar fovea sign" for defining ulnar wrist pain: an analysis of sensitivity and specificity. J Hand Surg Am 2007;32(4):438–44.

42. Glowacki KA, Shin LA. Stabilization of the unstable distal ulna: the Linscheid-Hui procedure. Tech Hand Up Extrem Surg 1999;3(4):229–36.

43. Millard GM, Budoff JE, Paravic V, et al. Functional bracing for distal radioulnar joint instability. J Hand Surg Am 2002;27(6):972–7.

44. O'Brien VH, Thurn J. A simple distal radioulnar joint orthosis. J Hand Ther 2013;26(3):287–90.

45. Nakamura T. Anatomical reattachment of the TFCC to the ulnar fovea using an ECU half-slip. J Wrist Surg 2015;4(1):15–21.

46. Adams BD, Berger RA. An anatomic reconstruction of the distal radioulnar ligaments for posttraumatic distal radioulnar joint instability. J Hand Surg Am 2002;27(2):243–51.

Treatment Options for Distal Radioulnar Joint Arthritis
Balancing Functional Demand and Bony Resection

Gina Farias-Eisner, MD[a], Stephen D. Zoller, MD[a], Nicholas Iannuzzi, MD[b],*

KEYWORDS

- DRUJ arthritis • Arthritis • Distal radioulnar joint • Instability • Arthroplasty • Prosthesis
- Ulnar-sided wrist pain • Triangular fibrocartilage complex

KEY POINTS

- The distal radioulnar joint is a diarthrodial articulation between the ulnar head and the sigmoid notch of the distal radius that permits forearm pronation and supination.
- The health of the articular cartilage relies heavily on the maintenance of correct joint alignment as afforded by the secondary distal radioulnar joint stabilizers and the triangular fibrocartilage complex.
- The goal of the history and examination are to establish the nature of the joint dysfunction in symptomatic patients and differentiate distal radioulnar joint arthritis from other causes of ulnar-sided wrist pain.
- Surgical options include resection arthroplasties and implant arthroplasties including ulnar head and total distal radioulnar joint arthroplasty.
- Selecting the best surgical intervention often means choosing the procedure with the set of disadvantages best suited for a specific patient.

INTRODUCTION

As humans have evolved, specific anatomic structures have developed that distinguish hominoids from other species. Although the size of the brain and the opposable thumb have, perhaps, received the most attention in anthropological literature, the distal radioulnar joint (DRUJ) may be of equal significance in defining humans' evolutionary advantage. Ed Almquist highlighted the importance of the DRUJ in humans' evolution in his review of the evolution of the DRUJ.

The dramatic difference in hominid evolution involved the size of the brain cavity and thus presumably the ability to control and use the highly developed tool, "the hand," with its freely movable wrist. The question posed by philosopher-anthropologists is whether this highly adaptic, most extraordinary instrument encouraged the brain to evolve to put it to better use, or vice versa.[1]

Despite its importance, the biomechanics and anatomy of the DRUJ were considered a mysterious "black box" until recently. Over the past

---

[a] Hand, Elbow & Shoulder Center at University of Washington Medical Center -Roosevelt, 4245 Roosevelt Way Northeast, Second Floor Seattle, WA 98105, USA; [b] Orthopaedic Surgery, Puget Sound VA, Department of Orthopaedics and Sports Medicine, Hand, Elbow & Shoulder Center at University of Washington Medical Center -Roosevelt, 4245 Roosevelt Way Northeast, Second Floor, Seattle, WA 98105, USA
* Corresponding author.
E-mail address: iannuzzi@uw.edu

Hand Clin 37 (2021) 575–586
https://doi.org/10.1016/j.hcl.2021.06.010
0749-0712/21/© 2021 Elsevier Inc. All rights reserved.

40 years, marked contributions have been made to the study of the anatomy, biomechanics, and pathophysiology of the DRUJ furthering our understanding and approach to reconstructive procedures.[2]

Hand surgeons have come to understand that the anatomic structures of the DRUJ are complex and work together to allow a combination of motion—both rotation and translation—and stability. Traumatic, congenital, inflammatory, and degenerative processes can disturb this sensitive balance and result in DRUJ arthritis—a challenging problem for the surgeon and patient alike. A variety of imperfect surgical solutions have been developed to address DRUJ arthritis, and each surgical technique has specific consequences. Because no perfect solution exists to address every patient with DRUJ arthritis, selecting the best surgical intervention often means choosing the procedure with the set of disadvantages best suited for a specific patient.

In this article, we discuss the anatomy and biomechanics of the DRUJ and the clinical approach to a patient with suspected DRUJ pathology. We also review the surgical treatment options for DRUJ arthritis, the expected outcomes of these procedures, and their respective shortcomings. It is our goal to provide an algorithm that prioritizes patient function with the goal of maintaining future therapeutic options.

DISTAL RADIOULNAR JOINT ARTHRITIS: ANATOMY AND BIOMECHANICS—A DELICATE EQUILIBRIUM OF STABILITY AND MOTION

The DRUJ is a diarthrodial articulation between the ulnar head and the sigmoid notch of the distal radius that permits forearm pronation and supination.[3,4] A shallow, concave articular surface, the sigmoid notch of the radius rotates around the seat of the fixed ulnar head. The sigmoid notch of the radius has an arc of curvature between 15 and 19 mm, which is nearly twice that of the ulnar head (8–10 mm)[5,6] (Fig. 1). This disparity in the radii of curvature creates an incongruity between the sigmoid notch and ulnar seat, permitting both rotational and translational motion within the DRUJ. In extremes of forearm rotation, the sigmoid notch is in contact with less than 10% of the ulnar head. Stable motion at the DRUJ is made possible by a combination of extrinsic and intrinsic stabilizers that provide both static and dynamic restraint across the joint.[7] As a result, compressive and shear forces are imparted on the DRUJ during pronosupination. The extrinsic stabilizers of the DRUJ consist of the semirigid extensor carpi ulnaris tendon sheath, the tension

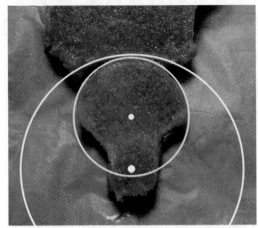

Fig. 1. Transverse section through the distal radius and ulna illustrating the sigmoid notch of the radius has an arc of curvature, which is nearly twice that of the ulnar head. The smaller, inner circle depicts the curvature of the ulnar head. The larger outer circle illustrates the curvature of the sigmoid notch. This disparity creates incongruity between the sigmoid notch and the ulnar seat permitting rotation and translational motion within the DRUJ. (*From* Hagert E, Hager CG Understanding stability of the distal radioulnar joint through an understanding of its anatomy. Hand Clin. 2010 Nov;26(4):459-66; with permission)

of the extensor carpi ulnaris as it crosses the head of the ulna, the dynamic support of the pronator quadratus, and the interosseous membrane of the forearm, including the distal oblique bundle of the interosseous membrane. Meanwhile, the triangular fibrocartilage complex (TFCC) provides intrinsic stabilization of the DRUJ and transmits load across the ulnocarpal joint.[2,4] The TFCC is a complex structure that includes the dorsal and palmar radioulnar ligaments, the ulnocarpal ligaments (including the ulnolunate and ulnotriquetral ligaments), the articular disk, the meniscus homologue, and the ECU tendon sheath.[8]

The sensory innervation of the DRUJ has also been described. In a series of cadaveric dissections, Hohenberger and colleagues[9] noted that the anterior interosseous nerve is responsible for a majority of the sensory innervation of the DRUJ. Articular branches of the anterior interosseous nerve are located distal to the proximal border of the pronator quadratus, between 4.8 and 6.2 cm proximal to the radial styloid for radii of 20.5 and 26.5 cm in length, respectively.[9] Interestingly, although denervation of the wrist may be performed for radiocarpal and midcarpal wrist pain with reasonably good results,[10,11] this procedure has not been described as a treatment option for DRUJ arthritis.

DISTAL RADIOULNAR JOINT ARTHRITIS: PATHOGENESIS

The health of the articular cartilage relies heavily on the maintenance of correct joint alignment as afforded by the secondary DRUJ stabilizers and the TFCC. Disrupting this delicate balance through trauma, inflammatory, and degenerative processes can result in DRUJ arthritis.

Incongruities of the articular surface owing to articular step-offs, malalignment of the distal radius after distal radius fractures, or distal ulnar fractures may alter the radio–ulnar contact area and lead to post-traumatic arthritis.[10,12] The reported prevalence of radiological post-traumatic arthritis of the radiocarpal or radioulnar joint after distal radius fractures varies in the literature and has been described as high as 65% after 6.7 years of follow-up.[13] In a systematic review analyzing the prevalence of radiological post-traumatic arthritis, Lameijer and colleagues[12] found that the prevalence of post-traumatic arthritis increased from 31% between 0 and 36 months after injury to 64% after more than 36 months after injury. The authors also noted that articular incongruity was a significant predictor for post-traumatic arthritis.[12] Distal radius fractures may also be complicated by DRUJ instability. Left untreated, instability at the DRUJ may alter the compressive and sheer forces across the joint, resulting in DRUJ arthritis.

The DRUJ is particularly susceptible to rheumatoid arthritis (RA). RA may cause cartilage degradation and synovial hypertrophy that may attenuate the synovial-lined ligamentous stabilizers that are critical to DRUJ stability.[14] Within 2 years of diagnosis, more than one-half of patients may have wrist pain and more than 90% may have wrist disease by 10 years.[15] The DRUJ is involved in 31% to 75% of these patients and is often the first compartment of the wrist involved.[16]

Osteoarthritis may develop in a relatively small population of patients as a result of manual activities or repetitive tasks. These patients may note pain with pronation and supination, decreased grip strength, crepitus, and difficulty performing activities of daily living.[17]

THE CLINIC PATIENT: DIAGNOSIS

Ulnar-sided wrist pain is often referred to as the "low back pain of the wrist" because its diagnosis and management may be difficult[18] (**Fig. 2**). The goals of the history and examination are to differentiate DRUJ arthritis from other causes of ulnar-sided wrist pain to establish the nature of the DRUJ dysfunction (**Fig. 3**).

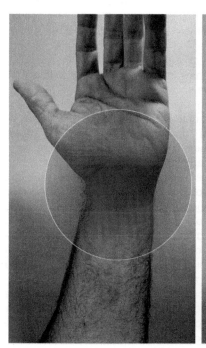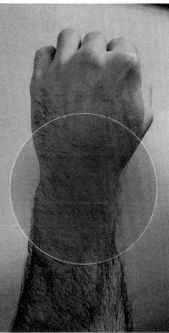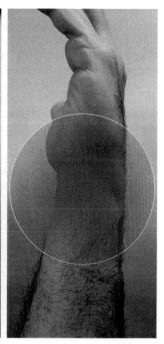

Fig. 2. Ulnar-sided wrist pain is often referred to as the "low back pain of the wrist" because of difficulties with diagnosis and management of the condition often presenting as vague wrist pain as illustrated elsewhere in this article. The goal of the history and examination are to establish the nature of the DRUJ dysfunction in symptomatic patients and differentiate DRUJ arthritis from other causes of ulnar-sided wrist pain.

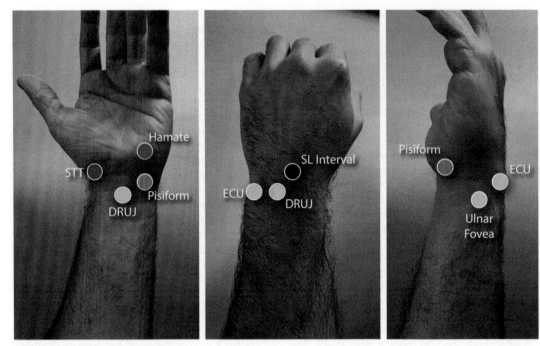

Fig. 3. A thorough examination through inspection, palpation, and provocative maneuvers of each of these intervals, focuses the differential diagnosis and allows the physician to differentiate DRUJ arthritis from other causes of ulnar-sided wrist pain. ECU, extensor carpi ulnaris; STT

Brogan and colleagues suggested using associated symptoms or findings to categorize patients experiencing ulnar-sided wrist pain.[7,11] Pain alone may result from ECU tendonitis or subluxation, a central TFCC tear, lunotriquetral ligament sprain, or pisotriquetral pathology.[7] Pain with instability may occur after avulsion of the deep distal radioulnar ligaments, a transverse tear of the ulnotriquetral and ulnolunate ligaments, extensor carpi ulnaris (ECU) subsheath tear, or a lunotriquetral ligament tear. Pain with arthritis may suggest ulnar impaction syndrome, pisotriquetral arthritis, or DRUJ arthritis.[7]

In approaching a patient with suspected DRUJ arthritis, attention should be paid to previous history of trauma and fractures involving the distal forearm as well as any past medical history involving RA. As mentioned elsewhere in this article, fractures about the DRUJ may result in incongruity of the articular surface or instability and lead to post-traumatic arthritis.[10] RA may result in synovitis of the DRUJ capsule and cause cartilage degradation, bony resorption, and instability.

Physical Examination

There are few physical examination maneuvers that specifically evaluate for DRUJ arthritis. Therefore, the physician should develop a standardized approach to ulnar-sided wrist pain that can

evaluate the multitude of potential diagnoses that may affect the ulnar side of the wrist. Examination of the DRUJ includes inspection, palpation, and provocative maneuvers (see **Fig. 3**). When evaluating the affected extremity, both wrists should be placed side by side with the contralateral wrist serving as a control. Particular attention should be directed to asymmetries, deformities, and prominence of the distal ulna.[19]

Inspection of the wrist may reveal a dorsal prominence of the ulnar head. Prominence that reduces with downward pressure but returns dorsally when released—the piano key sign—may be a marker of DRUJ instability. Dorsal prominence of the distal ulna may also represent caput ulnae syndrome, initially described in 1963 by the Swedish hand surgeon Magnus Backdahl. Caused by the pathologic changes of the DRUJ owing to RA, findings associated with caput ulnae syndrome include palmar subluxation and supination of the carpus, palmar subluxation of the ECU tendon, and a dorsally prominent ulnar head.[15] Patients with caput ulnae syndrome should also be evaluated for Vaughan–Jackson syndrome, or attritional rupture of the ulnar digital extension tendons caused by gliding of the tendons over the eroded ulnar head (**Fig. 4**).

Kleinman and colleagues[2] described stressing the TFCC by sitting opposite the patient with the patient's elbow on the examination table and the

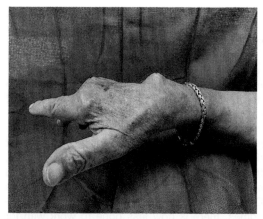

Fig. 4. Dorsal prominence of the distal ulna in a patient with caput ulnae syndrome.

fingers toward the ceiling. The patient's forearm is rotated into full supination, neutral, and full pronation, pushing the distal ulna toward the patient and pulling the radiocarpal unit toward the examiner through each position. Increased laxity compared with the contralateral side indicates DRUJ instability.[2]

The radioulnar compression test may elicit pain and crepitus, indicating DRUJ arthritis. During this maneuver, the examiner squeezes the distal ulna and distal radius together while the forearm is passively rotated. The examiner may note crepitus with rotation and patients may note increased pain with motion at the DRUJ.

A Brief Word on Imaging

Evaluation of the hand and wrist with radiography remains a mainstay when diagnosing arthritis of the DRUJ. Posteroanterior radiography of the wrist with the forearm in neutral rotation is helpful for the assessment of degenerative changes of the DRUJ and ulnar variance. Features of DRUJ arthritis radiographically are consistent with other forms of osteoarthritis, including a narrowing of the joint space, osteophytes, subchondral sclerosis, and subchondral cysts. Early radiographic signs of degenerative arthritis of the DRUJ typically occur in the proximal ulnar head and may spare the sigmoid notch. In the setting of RA, scalloping of the sigmoid notch may be present. A true lateral radiograph can demonstrate dorsal or volar displacement of the ulna, which may suggest instability. Contralateral imaging may be obtained to control for anatomic variants.[10]

Computed tomography (CT) scans depict the bony anatomy of the distal ulna and sigmoid notch at high resolution. Owing to the complex anatomy of the DRUJ, a CT scan should be obtained if DRUJ arthritis is suspected but is not clearly

evident on radiographs. A CT scan may also assist with preoperative planning as articular incongruities and the extent and location of osteophytes affecting the DRUJ may be better assessed with 3-dimensional imaging. Three-dimensional reconstructions of the DRUJ may facilitate this process. In the presence of small articular defects or osteophytes, less invasive procedures such as ulnar shortening osteotomy or limited resection could be considered, whereas more global joint abnormalities may prompt the surgeon to pursue more invasive procedures, including arthroplasty.

Suspected instability at the DRUJ may also be evaluated with CT scan. Amrami and colleagues described a method of evaluating instability in which the affected DRUJ is injected with anesthetic to ensure strength is not limited by pain. The patient enters the CT scanner in prone position and grips a device with the wrist in neutral, 60° of pronation, and 60° of supination. Axial images are taken in each position for evaluation of position of the ulna relative to the radius, and the contralateral side may be used as a control. The CT scans of the DRUJ in each position are evaluated for displacement of the ulnar head outside of the sigmoid notch.[10]

If concern persists for instability of the DRUJ or an incompetent TFCC, an MRI may be indicated. An MRI may be used to assess soft tissue components of the DRUJ and allow direct visualization of the ligaments associated with the DRUJ including the palmar and dorsal radioulnar ligaments, the ulnocarpal ligaments, and the TFCC. The absence of a functioning TFCC is a relative contraindication to a distal ulnar hemiresection and tendon interposition, as described by Bowers.

When the diagnosis of DRUJ arthritis remains unclear, intra-articular injection of lidocaine or lidocaine and a steroid may confirm the diagnosis. It may be useful to perform the DRUJ injection under fluoroscopic guidance using arthrography, because a large TFCC tear may allow lidocaine to enter the remainder of the wrist joint, limiting the diagnostic usefulness of the injection. Finally, diagnostic arthroscopy may be considered when other diagnostic tools have failed to provide a source of the patient's pain.[20]

Nonsurgical Options

The goals of nonsurgical management are (1) pain control with nonsteroidal anti-inflammatory drugs and intra-articular steroid injections, (2) preservation of joint function through a combination of activity modification, immobilization, and physical therapy, and (3) staving off surgery for as long as possible.

Intra-articular corticosteroid injections have been used to confirm diagnosis of DRUJ-related pain and may also be used to treat DRUJ disorders conservatively. Image guidance seems to improve the accuracy of injections, but not necessarily patient outcomes. In a randomized prospective single-blinded clinical study, Park and colleagues, evaluated the accuracy rate of ultrasound-guided versus palpation-guided intra-articular injections for the treatment of DRUJ disorders. Although ultrasound-guided intra-articular injections demonstrated significantly higher accuracy, there was no difference in clinical outcomes between the groups and all groups receiving injections demonstrated improved range of motion and Disabilities of the Arm, Shoulder, and Hand (DASH) scores.[21]

SURGICAL OPTIONS AND THEIR CONSEQUENCES—BONE AS CURRENCY

In formulating an operative plan for each patient, 2 issues are of particular interest to the clinician: the history of present illness and the demographic profile of the individual patient (age, occupation, hobbies, and medical comorbidities). By paying particular attention to these parameters, the patient and physician can anticipate the load that the DRUJ will be expected to bear over that patient's lifetime. Thus, the clinician can adapt a surgical plan tailored to the patient's needs (**Fig. 5**). Similar to nonsurgical options, the goal of surgical intervention is the (1) eradication of pain by eliminating articulation between the distal radius and

ulna, (2) preservation of joint function and stability, and (3) staving off future surgeries for as long as possible.

Surgical options comprise 2 main categories: resection arthroplasties and implant arthroplasties. As we present each surgical intervention and its shortcomings, it becomes apparent that in many ways bone is a form of currency. As discussed elsewhere in this article, DRUJ function relies on bony architecture and functioning soft tissue restraints. As bone at the DRUJ is resected, these soft tissue restraints may become lax and compromised. If the initial surgery to address DRUJ arthritis does not provide satisfactory outcomes, there is now less bone to work with for future surgeries, and either more extensive resection or implant arthroplasty may be required. Particularly in younger, higher demand patients, the surgeon should seek to optimize the patient's function and pain relief while preserving bone, and, consequently, future surgical options.

Limited Bony Resection: Options for the Low-Demand Patient

Limited resection techniques primarily developed in response to the complications associated with complete resection of the distal ulna as described by Darrach. The goal of these procedures is to maintain the TFCC and soft tissue stabilizers of the DRUJ while resecting the arthritic bone. The 2 procedures that fall into this category of treatment options include the hemiresection-interposition technique (HIT) as described by

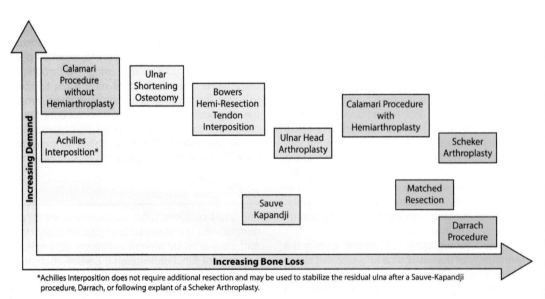

*Achilles Interposition does not require additional resection and may be used to stabilize the residual ulna after a Sauve-Kapandji procedure, Darrach, or following explant of a Scheker Arthroplasty.

Fig. 5. DRUJ options.

Bowers and the matched resection technique as described by Watson.

In 1985, Bowers described the HIT for DRUJ arthroplasty characterized by resection of the articular portion of the distal ulna with retention of the shaft and styloid with TFCC connections. Soft tissue was inserted into the resection cavity as a means for preventing convergence of the radius and ulna.[22] In Bowers' report, 71% of his 38 patients had RA. Following surgery, 85% had stable, painless pronation averaging 84° and 77° of supination.[22]

In a long-term outcome study assessing function, pain, and satisfaction scores in patients who had undergone HIT arthroplasty, Chen and colleagues found that patients with inflammatory arthritis had higher satisfaction and lower pain scores within their cohort, whereas men, older patients, and post-traumatic patients had higher pain scores, suggesting that HIT arthroplasty may be better suited for patients with inflammatory arthritis.[23]

The matched resection technique was first described by Watson. In 1985, Watson and colleagues[24] published their results reporting pain relief with relative preservation of DRUJ kinematics of the matched ulna resection in which the ulna is resected in a long sloping manner resembling an eccentrically sharpened pencil. The ulna is resected to optimize congruency with the sigmoid notch leaving the distal-most tip of the resected ulna.[24]

Despite attempts to preserve stability, studies have found that resection of the distal ulna disrupts DRUJ kinematics.[25] In a cadaveric study, Douglas and colleagues[26] demonstrated that, under neutral rotation, weighted and unweighted, matched hemiresection, and Darrach specimens demonstrated significant radioulnar convergence when compared with intact specimens, whereas DRUJ arthroplasty specimens demonstrated radioulnar convergence similar to intact specimens.

In an attempt to preserve stability, the Sauve–Kapandji fuses the ulnar head to the radius at the sigmoid notch and creates an osteotomy at the ulnar neck.[27] This procedure is often recommended for younger, high-demand patients.[20] The touted advantages of this procedure include limiting ulnar translocation and decreasing pain. In a retrospective review of patients who underwent Suave–Kapandji, QuickDASH scores demonstrated significant functional improvements after 1 year, and supination was significantly improved. However, postoperative complication rates were as high as 21% and commonly required hardware removal and revision osteotomies.[28] Other studies have discussed disadvantages of the Sauve–Kapandji procedure, including pseudoarthrosis and

nonunion, reossification of the bony gap, instability of the ulnar stump, and painful hardware.[29]

Limited Bony Resection: Options for the High-Demand Patient

Experience with the procedures discussed in this article has taught us that preservation of the DRUJ is important for a good clinical outcome in patients with early osteoarthritis. Scheker and colleagues[17] proposed ulnar shortening osteotomy as a technique to change the contact between the radial sigmoid notch and the ulnar head in patients with early DRUJ arthritis. In this prospective study, wrist rating scores based on pain, function status, range of motion, and grip, 7 of 32 were rated excellent, 11 of 32 were rated good, 9 of 32 were rated fair, and 5 of 32 were rated poor.[17] The mean lifting capacity was 7 kg postoperatively compared with 5 kg preoperatively.[17] This procedure is not recommended when cartilage at the DRUJ has been completely deteriorated, as in very advanced cases of osteoarthritis. However, it may be a good option in high-demand patients with no or limited instability and early DRUJ arthritis. Ulnar shortening osteotomy tightens the ligaments connecting the radioulnar and ulnocarpal joints, which may result not only in changes in the contact area, but also improve DRUJ stability.[30]

Complete Bony Resection: The Darrach Procedure

In 1912, the distal ulnar resection was described by Darrach for treatment of an irreducible DRUJ dislocation.[31] The Darrach procedure involves resection of the distal ulna with preservation of supporting soft tissue structures. Resection of the distal ulna may be considered in lower demand patients and may be appropriate when additional procedures, such as wrist arthrodesis or tendon reconstruction are planned for the same surgery, as may be the case in the setting of RA.

Although most often used in the setting of RA, Grawe and colleagues[32] described the Darrach procedure for DRUJ dysfunction with prior wrist trauma. The results seem encouraging demonstrating long-term follow-up (range, 6–20 years) with final average visual analog scale score for pain (0–4) and average wrist range of motion 85° and 78° and 41° and 45° for pronation/supination and flexion/extension, respectively. The authors concluded that the Darrach procedure can provide reliable good long-term outcomes for treatment of DRUJ pathology after a distal radius fracture. Although these results are promising, a large number of patients in the study were lost to follow-up,

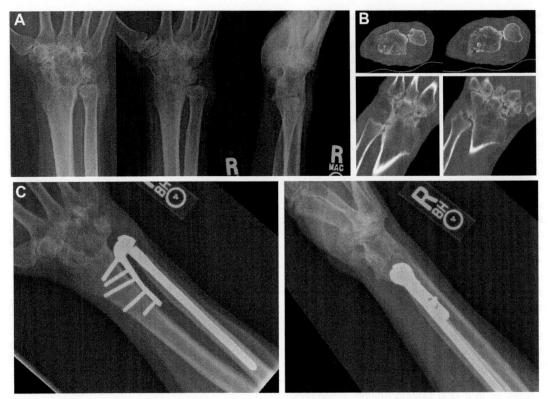

Fig. 6. (*A*) Right wrist anteroposterior, oblique, and lateral views demonstrating advanced DRUJ arthritis with evidence of sclerosis of the sigmoid notch and ulnar head, narrowing of the joint space and osteophytes of the ulnar head. (*B*) CT axial and coronal images of the right wrist demonstrating advanced DRUJ arthritis with evidence of sclerosis, subchondral cysts, and osteophytes of the sigmoid notch and ulnar head with loose bodies within the joint at the point of articulation with the ulnar head. (*C*) Right wrist anteroposterior and lateral images replacement of the ulnar head and sigmoid notch with total DRUJ arthroplasty.

leaving open the possibility that a number of patients could have had poor outcomes and sought treatment elsewhere.[32] Conversely, these patients may have had good outcomes for which they did not seek further follow-up.

The Darrach procedure has been demonstrated to improve the patient's pain, grip strength, and forearm motion.[33] Long-term complications including persistent pain and radioulnar dysfunction have been described.[34–36] Instability of the residual distal ulna and radioulnar impingement are some of the most common and severe consequences of the Darrach procedure. Contact between the resected distal ulna and radius may result in painful forearm rotation, crepitus, wrist instability, and weak grip.[37]

A variety of procedures and variations have been developed to mitigate symptoms associated with impingement. Zimmerman and colleagues[38] described their preferred method of the modified Darrach in which a radially inclined oblique osteotomy is made just proximal to the sigmoid notch to preserve the interosseous membrane, stabilize the

residual ulnar stump, and avoid a sharp subcutaneous prominence. The authors routinely stabilized the residual ulnar stump by splitting the ECU tendon in half longitudinally and securing a distally based slip of the ECU to the residual ulna.[38]

In patients with higher demand requirements, even when carefully executed as described elsewhere in this article, impingement may result between the distal ulna and radius. Papatheodorou and colleagues[37] described the interposition of an Achilles tendon allograft between the distal radius and the resected distal ulna. In a series of 27 patients with failed distal ulna resection with a mean age of 44 years, interposition arthroplasty with Achilles allograft resulted in grip strength improvement of 72% and total arc of forearm rotation improved an average of 69°.[37]

Arthroplasty

After any resection of the distal ulna, residual instability of the ulnar stump may cause pain during normal functional activities, especially with loading.[38,39] DRUJ arthroplasties have been designed to either replace an isolated ulnar head or act as a semiconstrained replacement of the entire DRUJ articulation.[40,41] By replacing resected portions of the DRUJ, arthroplasty options attempt to maintain normal DRUJ kinematics.

Ulnar Head Arthroplasty

Ulnar head replacement involves replacement of the arthritic, articular portion of the ulna while sparing the TFCC. Ulnar head arthroplasty indications include primary replacement of a degenerative ulnar head or salvage of ulnar stump instability following a Darrach or Sauve–Kapandji procedure.

Outcomes have been mixed. Sabo and colleagues[42] reported that although ulnar head arthroplasty has a high degree of satisfaction, it can leave a substantial degree of residual disability. Outcomes may also be highly variable based on the etiology of patient's disease. Patients with post-traumatic arthritis who underwent ulnar head arthroplasty tended to be less satisfied and rate their current disability higher than those who had arthroplasty either for inflammatory or osteoarthritic diagnoses.[42]

In a long-term series, with an average follow-up of 7.5 years, Axelsson and colleagues demonstrated improvement in supination, DASH score, and grip strength, and although full stability was not achieved, patients' pain resolved. Reports of metallic ulnar head implants have noted sigmoid fossa remodeling and bone resorption at the prosthesis collar with time.[43,44] In another series of ulnar head implants, Herzberg[45] evaluated bone resorption around the collar of the prosthesis and at the radial sigmoid notch. Bone resorption around the collar of the prosthesis was observed in 90% of 10 cases and radial sigmoid notch erosion opposite the implant was observed in 30% of cases at average follow-up of 36 months. In this group of patients, bone resorption occurred within the first postoperative year, then stabilized from 1 year to an average follow-up of 3 years.[45]

Owing to concerns regarding persistent pain and instability after ulnar head arthroplasty, Kakar and colleagues[46] developed a technique that combines partial ulnar head replacement with DRUJ interposition arthroplasty using a lateral meniscal allograft. In this procedure, the sigmoid notch is debrided and a lateral meniscal allograft is trimmed to match the size of the sigmoid notch. The purpose of this interposition is to decrease the contact area of the ulnar head with the surface of the sigmoid notch and deepen the concavity of the sigmoid notch to improve stability of the DRUJ.[46] In their series of 4 patients, the authors noted an increase in postoperative range of motion with an average increase in grip strength of 43%. All patients experienced marked decrease in their pain and no patients reported instability.[46] Resurfacing of the sigmoid notch using a meniscal allograft may decrease the amount of erosion of the sigmoid notch after ulnar head arthroplasty, although mid- and long-term data have not confirmed this possibility. Further study of this technique is warranted as this procedure may represent a viable surgical option for younger, more active patients with symptomatic DRUJ arthritis.

Total Distal Radioulnar Joint Arthroplasty

The Aptis DRUJ replacement prosthesis (Aptis Medical, Glenview, KY) consists of a semiconstrained implant designed to replace the function of the ulnar head, the sigmoid notch of the radius, and the TFC ligaments[47] (**Fig. 6**). The prosthesis allows longitudinal motion between the radius and ulna during pronation and supination of the forearm while reconstructing the ulnar articulation with the distal radius.[47]

Functional outcomes have overall been reported as positive, although a relatively high complication rate has been noted. In a retrospective review of 46 arthroplasties with the average patient age of 32 years, grip, lifting, DASH scores, and visual analog scale scores demonstrated statistically significant improvement after DRUJ replacement with a 5-year survival rate for the implant of 96%.[47]

In a retrospective review, DeGeorge and colleagues[48] evaluated 46 patients over 10 years and demonstrated that postoperative range of motion, grip strength, and visual analog scale pain scores were significantly improved compared with preoperative values after DRUJ arthroplasty. However, the overall complication rate was reported at 44.0% with complications noted in 22 of 50 arthroplasties. Major complications were identified in 8 of 50 wrists (16.0%) and minor ones in 20 of 50 wrists (40.0%). Eighteen operations were required to address complications in 8 patients.[48]

In a clinical series, evaluating complications of the Aptis device, Bellevue and colleagues[49] demonstrated 29% of patients required further surgery for complications, with the most common reason for surgery being periprosthetic fracture and infection.

SUMMARY

The DRUJ is a complex anatomic structure that allows for a combination of rotation and translation with extrinsic and intrinsic stabilizers that maintain stability through a delicate equilibrium. Traumatic, congenital, inflammatory, and degenerative processes can disturb this sensitive balance resulting in DRUJ arthritis. DRUJ arthritis is a challenging problem with no one-size-fits-all solution. When approaching the patient with DRUJ arthritis, we recommend understanding the functional demand of the individual patient and evaluating his or her soft tissue and bony integrity to implement patient-specific management. Selecting the best surgical intervention often means choosing the procedure with the set of complications and limitations best suited for the specific patient.

CASE PRESENTATION

Bowers made the observation that the best way to provide stability is to never lose it.[23] It is our opinion that, as bone at the DRUJ is resected, soft tissue restraints may become lax and compromised. We recommend that the surgeon seek to optimize the patient's function and pain relief while preserving bone, and, consequently, future surgical options, especially in high demand, young patients. We describe a case in which a modified Calamari[46] procedure was performed without distal ulna resection.

The patient, a 42 year-old special education teacher, sustained a wrist injury 2 years before presentation and underwent open TFCC repair with dorsal capsulorrhaphy at an outside institution. Upon presentation to our clinic, the patient complained of ongoing ulnar-sided wrist pain exacerbated by forearm pronation and supination, with tenderness and crepitus localized to the DRUJ. Radiographs revealed sclerosis and osteophytes in the sigmoid notch as well as irregularity of the ulnar head with DRUJ joint space narrowing (**Fig. 7**A–C). Given the demands of her occupation and young age, the patient wished to avoid prosthetic arthroplasty. We therefore elected to perform a lateral meniscus interpositional

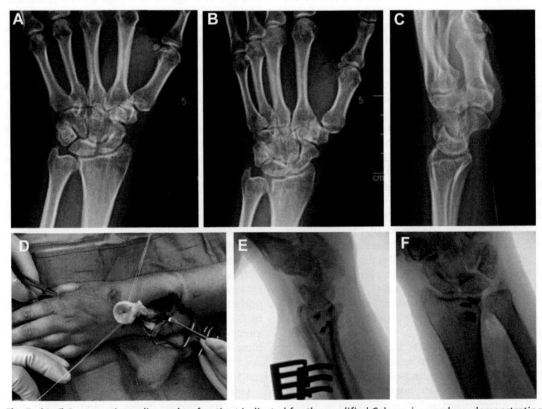

Fig. 7. (*A–C*) Preoperative radiographs of patient indicated for the modified Calamari procedure, demonstrating sigmoid notch sclerosis and osteophytes, irregularity of ulnar head, and narrowing of DRUJ space. (*D*) Intraoperative photo demonstrating 9'o clock, 12 o'clock, and 3 o'clock suture anchors and corresponding sutures to reduce meniscal allograft to sigmoid notch, with ulnar head intact. (*E, F*) Intraoperative fluoroscopy demonstrating placement of suture anchors (the proximal most suture anchor was not used for this procedure).

arthroplasty in the manner of Kakar and colleagues, modified to preserve the ulnar head.

Under tourniquet control, a longitudinal incision was made over the fifth extensor compartment, and the retinaculum overlying the fifth compartment was divided. The extensor digiti quinti was transposed dorsally and radially. A trapezoidal ulnar-based flap of the dorsal wrist capsule was then created, protecting the ECU tendon. To dislocate the ulnar head dorsally, the dorsoradial insertion of the TFCC on the radius was released, preserving its ulnar insertion. A lamina spreader was inserted proximal to the DRUJ to sublux and separate the ulnar head, permitting access to the sigmoid notch. Three 2.7-mm Arthrex corkscrew suture anchors (Arthrex, Naples, FL) were placed in the sigmoid notch, at 9 o'clock, 12 o'clock, and 3 o'clock, leaving the proximal 6 o'clock space free. The lateral meniscus was then prepared in the manner of Kakar and colleagues,[46] and the meniscal allograft was reduced to the sigmoid notch via 2.0 permanent braided suture from the anchors (see **Fig. 7**D–F). The distal 12 o'clock suture was also used to repair the dorsoradial limb of the TFCC and dorsal capsule. The wrist was ranged through pronation and supination, with elimination of crepitus. Postoperatively, the wrist was immobilized in supination for 6 weeks followed by gentle progression of range of motion exercises under hand therapist guidance.

DISCLOSURE

The authors have nothing to disclose.

REFERENCES

1. Almquist EE. Evolution of the distal radioulnar joint. Clin Orthop Relat Res 1992;275:5–13.
2. Kleinman WB. Stability of the distal radioulnar joint: biomechanics, pathophysiology, physical diagnosis, and restoration of function what we have learned in 25 years. J Hand Surg Am 2007;32(7):1086–106.
3. Af Ekenstam F. Anatomy of the distal radioulnar joint. Clin Orthop Relat Res 1992;275:14–8.
4. Huang J, Hanel D. Anatomy and Biomechanics of the Distal Radioulnar Joint. Hand Clin 2012;28(2):157–63.
5. Af Ekenstam F, Hagert CG. Anatomical studies on the geometry and stability of the distal radio ulnar joint. Scand J Plast Reconstr Surg 1985;19:17–25.
6. Tolat AR, Stanley JK, Trail IA. A cadaveric study of the anatomy and stability of the distal radioulnar joint in the coronal and transverse planes. J Hand Surg Br 1996;21:587–94.
7. Brogan D, Berger R, Kakar S. Ulnar-sided Wrist Pain A Critical Analysis Review. JBJS Rev 2019;7(5):e1.
8. Nakamura T. Arthroscopic management of ulnar pain. Springer; 2012. p. 15–23.
9. Hohenberger GM, Maier MJ, Dolcet C, et al. Sensory Nerve Supply of the Distal Radio-Ulnar Joint with Regard to Wrist Denervation. J Hand Surg Eur Vol 2017;42(6):586–91.
10. Faucher G, Zimmerman R, Zimmerman N. Instability and arthritis of the distal radioulnar joint: a critical analysis review. JBJS Rev 2016;4(12):e3.
11. Amarami K, Moran S, Berger R, et al. Imaging of the distal radioulnar joint. Hand Clin 2010;467–75.
12. Lameijer DM, Duis HJ, Van Dusseldrop I, et al. Prevalence of posttraumatic arthritis and the association with outcome measures following distal radius fractures in non-osteoporotic patients: a systematic review. Arch Orthop Trauma Surg 2017;137(11):1499–513.
13. Knirk JL, Jupiter JB. Intra-articular fractures of the distal end of the radius in young adults. J Bone Joint Surg Am 1986;68(5):647–59.
14. Lee S, Hauseman M. Management of the distal radioulnar joint in rheumatoid arthritis. Hand Clin 2005;21(4):577–89.
15. Rizzo M, Cooney W. Current concepts for the rheumatoid wrist. Hand Clin 2011;27(1):57–72.
16. De Smet L. The distal radioulnar join in rheumatoid arthritis. Acta Orthop Belg 2006;72(4):381–6.
17. Scheker LR, Severo A. Ulnar Shortening for the Treatment of Early Post-Traumatic Osteoarthritis at the Distal Radioulnar Joint. J Hand Surg Br 2001;26(1):41–4.
18. Ahn AK, Chang D, Plate AM. Triangular fibrocartilage complex tears: a review. Bull NYU Hosp Jt Dis 2006;64:114–8.
19. Kakar S, Garcia-Elias M. The "four-leaf clover" treatment algorithm: a practical approach to manage disorders of the distal radioulnar joint. J Hand Surg Am 2016;41(4):551–64.
20. Low CK, Chew WYC. Results of Sauve-Kapandji procedure. Singapore Med J 2002;43(3):135–7.
21. Nam SH, Kim J, Lee JH, et al. Palpation versus ultrasound-guided corticosteroid injections and short-term effect in the distal radioulnar joint disorder: a randomized, prospective single-blinded study. Clin Rheumatol 2014;33(12):1807–14.
22. Bowers WH. Distal radioulnar joint arthroplasty: the hemiresection-interposition technique. J Hand Surg Am 1985;10(2):169–78.
23. Nawijn F, Verhiel S, Jupiter JB, et al. Hemiresection interposition arthroplasty of the distal radioulnar joint: a long-term outcome study. Hand (N Y) 2019. https://doi.org/10.1177/1558944719873430. 1558944719873430.
24. Watson HK, Gabuzda GM. Matched distal ulna resection for posttraumatic disorders of the DRUJ. J Hand Surg Am 1992;17(4):724–30.
25. Shaaban H, Giakas G, Bolton M, et al. The distal radioulnar joint as a load-bearing mechanism—a

biomechanical study. J Hand Surg Am 2004;29(1): 85–95.

26. Douglas KC, Parks BG, Tsai MA, et al. The biomechanical stability of salvage procedures for distal radioulnar joint arthritis. J Hand Surg Am 2014;39(7): 1274–9.

27. Houdek MT, Wagner ER, Moran SL, et al. Disorders of the distal radioulnar joint. Plast Reconstr Surg 2015;135(1):161–72.

28. Giberson-Chen C, Leland HA, Benavent KA, et al. Functional outcomes after Sauve-Kapandji arthrodesis. J Hand Surg Am 2020;45(5):408–16.

29. Carter PB, Stuart PR. The Sauve-Kapandji procedure for posttraumatic disorders of the distal radioulnar joint. J Bone Joint Surg Br 2000;82(7):1013–8.

30. Nishiwaki M, Nakamura T, Nakao Y, et al. Ulnar shortening effect on distal radioulnar joint stability: a biomechanical study. J Hand Surg Am 2005; 30(4):719–26.

31. Lau FH, Chung KC. William Darrach, MD: his life and his contribution to hand surgery. J Hand Surg Am 2006;31(7):1056–60.

32. Grawe B, Heincelman C, Stern P. Functional results for the Darrach procedure: a long-term outcome study. J Hand Surg Am 2012;37(12):2475–80.

33. Tulipan DJ, Eaton EF, Eberhar RE. The Darrach procedure defended: technique redefined and long-term follow-up. J Hand Surg Am 1991;16(3):438–44.

34. Field J, Majkowski RJ, Leslie IJ. Poor results of Darrach's procedure after wrist injuries. J Bone Joint Surg Br 1993;75(1):53–7.

35. Sauerbier M, Berger RA, Fujita M, et al. Radioulnar convergence after distal ulnar resection: mechanical performance of two commonly used soft tissue stabilizing procedures. Acta Orthop Scand 2003;74(4):420–8.

36. McKee MD, Richards RR. Dynamic radio-ulnar convergence after the Darrach procedure. J Bone Joint Surg Br 1996;78(3):413–8.

37. Papatheodorou LK, Rubright JH, Kokkalis ZT, et al. Resection interposition arthroplasty for failed distal ulna resections. J Wrist Surg 2013;2(1):13–8.

38. Zimmerman RM, Jupiter JB. Instability of the distal radioulnar joint. J Hand Surg Eur 2014;39:727–38.

39. Moulton LS, Giddins GEB. Distal radio-ulnar implant arthroplasty: a systematic review. J Hand Surg Eur Vol 2017;42E(8):827–38.

40. Berger RA, Cooney WP. Use of an ulnar head endo-prosthesis for treatment of an unstable distal ulnar resection: review of mechanics, indications, and surgical technique. Hand Clin 2005;21:603–20.

41. Scheker LR. Implant arthroplasty for the distal radioulnar joint. J Hand Surg Am 2008;33:1639–44.

42. Sabo MT, Talwalkar S, Hayton M, et al. Intermediate outcomes of ulnar head arthroplasty. J Hand Surg Am 2014;39(12):2405–11.e1.

43. Van Schoonhoven J, Fernandez DL, Bowers WH, et al. Salvage of failed resection arthroplasties of the distal radio-ulnar joint using a new ulnar head prosthesis. J Hand Surg Am 2000;25:438–46.

44. Willis AA, Berger RA, Cooney WP. Arthroplasty of the DRUJ using a new ulnar head endoprosthesis: preliminary report. J Hand Surg Am 2007;32:177–89.

45. Herzberg G. Periprosthetic bone resorption and sigmoid notch erosion around ulnar head implants: a concern? Hand Clin 2010;26(4):573–7.

46. Kakar S, Noureldin M, Elhassan B. Ulnar head replacement and sigmoid notch resurfacing arthroplasty with a lateral meniscal allograft: 'calamari procedure'. J Hand Surg Eur Vol 2017;42(6): 567–72.

47. Rampazzo A, Gharb BB, Brock G, et al. Functional outcomes of the AptiseScheker distal radioulnar joint replacement in patients under 40 years old. J Hand Surg Am 2015;40(7):1397–403.

48. DeGeorge BR Jr, Berger RA, Shin AY. Constrained implant arthroplasty for distal radioulnar joint arthrosis: evaluation and management of soft tissue complications. J Hand Surg Am 2019;44(7):614. e1–9.

49. Bellevue KD, Thayer MD, Pouliot M, et al. Complications of semiconstrained distal radioulnar joint arthroplasty. J Hand Surg Am 2018;43(6):566.e1–9.

UNITED STATES POSTAL SERVICE ®

Statement of Ownership, Management, and Circulation
(All Periodicals Publications Except Requester Publications)

1. Publication Title	2. Publication Number		3. Filing Date
HAND CLINICS	000 – 709		9/18/2021

4. Issue Frequency	5. Number of Issues Published Annually	6. Annual Subscription Price
FEB, MAY, AUG, NOV	4	$439.00

7. Complete Mailing Address of Known Office of Publication (Not printer) (Street, city, county, state, and ZIP+4®)

ELSEVIER INC.
230 Park Avenue, Suite 800
New York, NY 10169

Contact Person
Malathi Samayan

Telephone (Include area code)
91-44-4299-4507

8. Complete Mailing Address of Headquarters or General Business Office of Publisher (Not printer)

ELSEVIER INC.
230 Park Avenue, Suite 800
New York, NY 10169

9. Full Names and Complete Mailing Addresses of Publisher, Editor, and Managing Editor (Do not leave blank)

Publisher (Name and complete mailing address)

Dolores Meloni, ELSEVIER INC.
1600 JOHN F KENNEDY BLVD. SUITE 1800
PHILADELPHIA, PA 19103-2899

Editor (Name and complete mailing address)

LAUREN BOYLE, ELSEVIER INC.
1600 JOHN F KENNEDY BLVD. SUITE 1800
PHILADELPHIA, PA 19103-2899

Managing Editor (Name and complete mailing address)

PATRICK MANLEY, ELSEVIER INC.
1600 JOHN F KENNEDY BLVD. SUITE 1800
PHILADELPHIA, PA 19103-2899

10. Owner (Do not leave blank. If the publication is owned by a corporation, give the name and address of the corporation immediately followed by the names and addresses of all stockholders owning or holding 1 percent or more of the total amount of stock. If not owned by a corporation, give the names and addresses of the individual owners. If owned by a partnership or other unincorporated firm, give its name and address as well as those of each individual owner. If the publication is published by a nonprofit organization, give its name and address.)

Full Name	Complete Mailing Address
WHOLLY OWNED SUBSIDIARY OF REED/ELSEVIER, US HOLDINGS	1600 JOHN F KENNEDY BLVD. SUITE 1800 PHILADELPHIA, PA 19103-2899

11. Known Bondholders, Mortgagees, and Other Security Holders Owning or Holding 1 Percent or More of Total Amount of Bonds, Mortgages, or Other Securities. If none, check box ▸ ☐ None

Full Name	Complete Mailing Address
N/A	

12. Tax Status (For completion by nonprofit organizations authorized to mail at nonprofit rates) (Check one)
The purpose, function, and nonprofit status of this organization and the exempt status for federal income tax purposes:
☒ Has Not Changed During Preceding 12 Months
☐ Has Changed During Preceding 12 Months (Publisher must submit explanation of change with this statement)

PS Form 3526, July 2014 (Page 1 of 4 (see instructions page 4)) PSN: 7530-01-000-9931 PRIVACY NOTICE: See our privacy policy on www.usps.com.

---

13. Publication Title	14. Issue Date for Circulation Data Below
HAND CLINICS	MAY 2021

15. Extent and Nature of Circulation			Average No. Copies Each Issue During Preceding 12 Months	No. Copies of Single Issue Published Nearest to Filing Date
a. Total Number of Copies (Net press run)			304	280
b. Paid Circulation (By Mail and Outside the Mail)	(1)	Mailed Outside-County Paid Subscriptions Stated on PS Form 3541 (Include paid distribution above nominal rate, advertiser's proof copies, and exchange copies)	186	169
	(2)	Mailed In-County Paid Subscriptions Stated on PS Form 3541 (Include paid distribution above nominal rate, advertiser's proof copies, and exchange copies)	0	0
	(3)	Paid Distribution Outside the Mails Including Sales Through Dealers and Carriers, Street Vendors, Counter Sales, and Other Paid Distribution Outside USPS®	88	82
	(4)	Paid Distribution by Other Classes of Mail Through the USPS (e.g. First-Class Mail®)	0	0
c. Total Paid Distribution (Sum of 15b (1), (2), (3), and (4))		▸	274	251
d. Free or Nominal Rate Distribution (By Mail and Outside the Mail)	(1)	Free or Nominal Rate Outside-County Copies included on PS Form 3541	13	12
	(2)	Free or Nominal Rate In-County Copies Included on PS Form 3541	0	0
	(3)	Free or Nominal Rate Copies Mailed at Other Classes Through the USPS (e.g. First-Class Mail)	0	0
	(4)	Free or Nominal Rate Distribution Outside the Mail (Carriers or other means)	13	12
e. Total Free or Nominal Rate Distribution (Sum of 15d (1), (2), (3) and (4))		▸	13	12
f. Total Distribution (Sum of 15c and 15e)		▸	287	263
g. Copies not Distributed (See Instructions to Publishers #4 (page #3))		▸	17	17
h. Total (Sum of 15f and g)		▸	304	280
i. Percent Paid (15c divided by 15f times 100)		▸	95.47%	95.43%

☒ If you are claiming electronic copies, go to line 16 on page 3. If you are not claiming electronic copies, skip to line 17 on page 3.

16. Electronic Copy Circulation		Average No. Copies Each Issue During Preceding 12 Months	No. Copies of Single Issue Published Nearest to Filing Date
a. Paid Electronic Copies	▸		
b. Total Paid Print Copies (Line 15c) + Paid Electronic Copies (Line 16a)	▸		
c. Total Print Distribution (Line 15f) + Paid Electronic Copies (Line 16a)	▸		
d. Percent Paid (Both Print & Electronic Copies) (16b divided by 16c × 100)	▸		

☒ I certify that 50% of all my distributed copies (electronic and print) are paid above a nominal price.

17. Publication of Statement of Ownership

☒ If the publication is a general publication, publication of this statement is required. Will be printed ☐ Publication not required.

in the November 2021 issue of this publication.

18. Signature and Title of Editor, Publisher, Business Manager, or Owner

Malathi Samayan

Malathi Samayan - Distribution Controller

Date 9/18/2021

I certify that all information furnished on this form is true and complete. I understand that anyone who furnishes false or misleading information on this form or who omits material or information requested on the form may be subject to criminal sanctions (including fines and imprisonment) and/or civil sanctions (including civil penalties).

PS Form 3526, July 2014 (Page 2 of 4) PRIVACY NOTICE: See our privacy policy on www.usps.com.

Moving?

Make sure your subscription moves with you!

To notify us of your new address, find your **Clinics Account Number** (located on your mailing label above your name), and contact customer service at:

Email: journalscustomerservice-usa@elsevier.com

800-654-2452 (subscribers in the U.S. & Canada)
314-447-8871 (subscribers outside of the U.S. & Canada)

Fax number: 314-447-8029

Elsevier Health Sciences Division
Subscription Customer Service
3251 Riverport Lane
Maryland Heights, MO 63043

*To ensure uninterrupted delivery of your subscription, please notify us at least 4 weeks in advance of move.

Printed and bound by CPI Group (UK) Ltd, Croydon, CR0 4YY

08/05/2025

01864700-0013